CW00866455

31

To Margaret.

Hope you enjoy,

Tricia ☺

The Scar that Won't Heal.

Stress, Trauma and Unresolved Emotion in Chronic Disease

The Science and Practice of Recovery

By Patricia Worby, MSc, PhD*

Text © Patricia Worby, 2015

The moral rights of the author have been asserted.

All rights reserved. No part of this book may be reproduced by any mechanical, photographic or electronic process, or in the form of a phonographic recording; nor may it be stored in a retrieval system, transmitted or otherwise be copied for public or private use, other than for 'fair use' as brief quotations embodied in articles and reviews, without prior written permission of the publisher.

The information given in this book is for information purposes only and should not be treated as a substitute for professional medical advice; always consult a medical practitioner. Any use of information in this book is at the reader's discretion and risk and should be under the direction of a competent physician or qualified medical professional. Neither the author nor the publisher can be held responsible for any loss, claim or damage arising out of the use, or misuse, of the suggestions made, the failure to take medical advice or for any material on third party websites.

A catalogue record for this book is available from the British Library.

ISBN-13: 978-1517558925
ISBN-10: 1517558921

CONTENTS

ACKNOWLEDGEMENTS

No book writes itself, though the best ones are given to us in inspiration. I was inspired to write this book by the many clients who have come through my door, ostensibly to be helped and hopefully healed but who have then, in the process, given me such learning and led me to further new ideas and investigations. I wish to thank them (and they know who they are) and my friends and family who have been willing to discuss these ideas openly with me. In particular; my partner Jill, who continues to inspire me with her willingness to work through our vulnerabilities and her dedication to improving the educational experience of international students, my brother Allan who, though he 'suffered' through the same childhood which left us disconnected from each other, has come through as my friend and confidant... And of course my Mum and Dad who did their best and for whom I have developed an overdue respect. Although all of us have a different language with which to express ourselves, more often than not these days, there is at least some dialogue and sometimes connection.

I wish to thank all the colleagues who helped me along the way, Adam Eason for his book writing course which allowed me to begin the process (always the hardest part), Alison Adams for showing me the way via her brilliant book and giving me so many great links to help in the process of publishing, to Sue Warren for her valiant proof-reading and correcting my occasionally unclear expressions and Elaine Wilkins and the great team at the Chrysalis Effect who mentored me in my new career. I wish also to highlight the work of others in the field of trauma therapy - those I know of: Dr Janina Fisher and Carolyn Spring of the survivor group PODS whose trainings I completed and which changed my understanding, Bessel van der Kolk, whose book 'The Body Keeps the Score' came out just as I was starting to write mine which raised the bar, Uri Bergmann whose book on the Neurobiological foundations of EMDR pre-empted my own, Brené Brown whose work on shame and vulnerability underscores my work with clients, and the numerous other wonderful authors, therapists and researchers who continue to help us understand ourselves better.

My book is naturally imperfect (not a bad thing), but it is heartfelt and born out of experience. Any errors or omissions are mine alone but I hope it adds to the study of vulnerability of the human experience in a way that moves us on towards a more compassionate society. Mental ill health is increasingly common and linked to the chronic illnesses of the body in ways which we are only now beginning to discover. Trauma as the root of that ill health is largely ignored and misunderstood by both public policy makers and health professionals. It is hoped that this book will add to the pressure to change the way we view health and illness so that fewer people have to suffer the confusion and despair that I did in my journey to recovery.

FOREWORD

At last, a fascinating and compelling work revealing the insidious nature of early trauma and its impact on the nation's health. I believe Patricia's work is a must read for health professionals providing solid argument for the cultural shift required to oust the current model of healthcare in the western world. It not only exposes the folly of routinely prescribing drugs to numb emotional and physical pain but offers solid, healthy alternatives. This author provides us with detailed and concrete science yet manages to touch the soul with deeply personal accounts of childhood experiences that will create a multitude of 'light bulb moments' in the reader. A superbly influential book.

Elaine Wilkins, Founder and Director of the Chrysalis Effect, the UK's only CFS/ME and Fibromyalgia Online Recovery Programme.

By the same author

The 7 Keys to Unlocking your Energy   available free on the website

www.alchemytherapies.co.uk

GLOSSARY OF TECHNICAL TERMS
(*first mentions in the text are in bold*).

Adrenaline (Epinephrine in the US) – principle hormone of the stress response responsible for raising the heart rate and preparing the muscles for action.

Adenosine di-phosphate (ADP) – the energy molecule of the cell (reduced form with two phosphates attached).

Adenosine tri-phosphate (ATP) - the energy molecule of the cell (oxidised form with three phosphates attached).

Afferent nerve fibres – travel towards the brain

Allostasis is the process of achieving stability, or homeostasis, through physiological or behavioral change

Amgydala – the almond-shaped part of the brain's limbic system that senses threat

Amino acid - the building blocks of proteins

ANS - Autonomic nervous system – the part of the nervous system responsible for automatic actions like breathing, heart rate, etc. Happens without conscious control

Anterior cingulate cortex (ACC) – the filtering system of the brain

Bioluminescence – the ability of living things especially DNA to emit photons at a range invisible to the human eye. Potentially containing information.

Catastrophising – an NLP term that describes the act of constructing a worst case scenario from past experience, one of the many cognitive distortions we make routinely.

Cell Danger Response (CDR) – a failure of the mitochondrial energy pathway due to various causes; toxins, stress and illness.

CFS/ME – Chronic Fatigue Syndrome or **Myalgic Encephalopathy** – a disease characterised by severe fatigue following mental or physical activity. It shares a lot of the same symptoms with Fibromyalgia except the dominant symptom is fatigue not pain.

Corticotrophic releasing hormone CRH - released by the hypothalamus to signal the beginning of the stress response in the HPA axis

Central nervous system (CNS) –. The brain and spinal cord which along with the peripheral nervous system forms the basis of our interaction with the sensory world.

Codon – a triplet of bases ('letters') in the backbone of the DNA molecule which codes for an amino acid (the building block of proteins).

Corpus callosum (CC) – a bunch of fibres between the left and right hemispheres which controls cross-talk (dialogue) between the two.

Detoxification - the process of keeping the blood free of toxins by the liver, including the by-products of pharmaceutical drug breakdown and endogenous toxins from food and other ingested/ inhaled, or absorbed chemicals. Is a two-stage sequence of enzymatic reactions.

Efferent – nerve fibres which travel from the brain

Electron Transport Chain (ETC) – sequence of molecules on the inner membrane of a mitochondrion that produces energy for the cell.

Emotional Freedom Technique (EFT) – a psychosensory therapy also called Meridian tapping involving a sequence of taps on the body whilst feeling the problem and stating acceptance. Clears traumatically stored procedural memories in the limbic system.

Evidence-based medicine (EBM) is the 'gold standard' of care in Western medicine and seeks to only use treatments or interventions that have been thoroughly tested in Randomised Control Trials (RCT). These laboratory based studies demonstrate effects of the treatment compared to a placebo (usually a sham / or no treatment). Works well when comparing a drug against a placebo pill but almost impossible when looking at more complex interventions such as nutrition or lifestyle change as there are many confounding factors. Often excludes other observational evidence.

Fibromyalgia – formerly called fibrositis is a disease characterised by intense muscle pain in certain segments of the body (usually back neck and shoulders) that is unrelieved by rest. It has concomitant issues of fatigue and brain fog, dizziness and shares a lot of the symptoms of ME or CFS to which it is linked functionally.

Functional MRI (fMRI) a form of magnetic resonance imaging that allows one to view processes happening in real time; useful for studying which areas of the brain light up during different tasks.

Glycolysis – the anaeorobic (without oxygen) energy generating pathway of the cell

Heart Rate Variability (HRV) – the difference between heart beats plotted against time as a measure of health of the autonomic nervous system.

Hippocampus – part of the limbic system that date stamps events and stores them as memories in the past.

Hypoarousal – a dissociative response where the dorsal vagal parasympathetic nerve is in charge. Characterised by freeze and fatigue

Hypothalamus - Pituitary - Adrenal system or **HPA axis** –the interconnected 3 part system of brain and endrocrine organs that communicates and activates the stress response

Interoception - the signals the brain receives from internal processes like heart rate, blood pressure and pH. These must be monitored carefully for healthy functioning.

Limbic System – the mammalian or 'emotional brain' consisting of: **thalamus** (relay station), **hypothalamus** (threat evaluator), **hippocampus** (date stamp and our normal memory processing centre), and the **amygdala**, the brain's "fire alarm" and smoke detector.

Long term potentiation (LTP) – the ability of neural networks in the brain to become more efficient the more often they fire; breeds habits of thinking and behaviour

Memory consolidation – the pattern of neural networks that fired at the time of a particular event are stored so that by re-firing these networks the memory is 'stored'.

Mirror neurons - neuron (nerve cells) that allow us to notice and respond to facial and bodily signals.

Mutations - errors in the replication and transcription (reading) of DNA which are damaging to the organism as the proteins produced do not function properly.

Mitochondriopathy – failure of the mitochondria as the basis of disease.

Neuro linguistic programming (NLP) – a model of interpersonal communication using the relationship between brain behaviour (neuro) via language (linguistic) to influence successful patterns of behaviour (programming)

Neuroplasticity – how the brain adapts to its environment by building new nerve connections to make the process more energy efficient and more automatic.

Nocioceptor – a noxious stimulus receptor in the peripheral nervous system which transmits damage signals up the sensory nerve fibres

 Noradrenaline – a neurotransmitter produced by the brain which is the equivalent of the adrenaline in the adrenals; fires up the stress response to help memories be retained.

Persistent (chronic) pain – pain that has been ongoing for more than 3 months usually as a result of over sensitisation of pain response in the brain.

Raynaud's syndrome (a hyper-reactivity of the vessels in the extremities (usually the fingers) causing blood flow to be restricted – sometimes called 'white finger' for that reason

Scleroderma, a potentially serious auto-immune condition which involves over-production of collagen in the skin and elsewhere which can be fatal if it affects the internal organs

Spindle cells - specialised thickened nerve fibres providing an interface between thoughts and emotions by integrating information from existing neural pathways allowing you to make quick leaps in understanding.

Somatisation - feeling emotions through the body rather than as feelings

Subjective Units of Distress (SUD) - is a self-rating scale from 1-10 that a client will use both to rate the intensity of a problem and to mark progress when (hopefully) it lowers as treatment progresses. Often used in Psychosensory therapies.

Synapse - gap between neurons

T3 (triiodothyronine) thyroid hormone with three iodine molecules attached - active

T4 (thyroxine) thyroid hormone with four iodine molecules – inactive

Tension Myoneural Syndrome (TMS) – John Sarno's term for the process of emotional causation of physical pain via an overactive nervous system of 'fight, flight and freeze' causing oxygen deprivation and lactic acid formation within the nerves or muscles = 'centralised pain' or 'psychogenic pain' in other models.

PROLOGUE

I never imagined I'd be where I am now. As a teenager I had very clear views on the kind of person I'd be by the time I was grown up. I'd be a famous scientist who found the cure for cancer, or something of that sort. The career choices moved around a bit; sometimes I imagined being a doctor (but I knew I'd never cope with the competitiveness of medical training) or perhaps a great teacher – at the very least someone 'making a difference'. I never imagined I'd have to go through the sometimes painful experiences I've been through but, somehow, I've got here.

I now work as a Mindbody[1] therapist specialising in releasing trauma and unresolved emotions. It is often said that therapists are often people who have suffered in some way themselves and the therapy they choose is frequently the one they most need! In fact, at a conference for trauma therapists I attended recently, the speaker, Bessel van der Kolk did a straw poll of therapists in the room who had experienced trauma themselves and about two thirds of hands went up! People are drawn to do what they needed when they were suffering. It could be considered a form of 're-enactment' (which I cover later) and hearing another's trauma story is a way of healing ourselves. Luckily there are tools around now which minimise re-traumatisation and rely less and less on telling the story.

Why then have I chosen to tell you mine? In this book I want to introduce you to the understanding I have reached about myself and trauma is a big part of the story. I had no ambition or plans to work in this area until a few years ago when my first trauma client came to see me. This lady so perplexed and horrified me with her story and the symptoms she was suffering I knew I had to find out what was going on. Since that first client, I got another and then another. Each story subtly different but also with striking similarities.

I had to ask myself - why me? What is it about me that attracts this type of client? I wasn't advertising as a trauma therapist. I was a newly qualified massage therapist having just started a new career in my 40's after searching for something that would inspire me and enable me to work with my hands as well as my heart. I had no inkling of what was in store for me. I can look back now and smile to myself as it's quite clear that the universe/ god/ fate (choose your theology) had clear plans for me. I was to find, time and time again, that trauma lay at the heart of so many of my clients' symptoms and I was led, sometimes gently, sometimes kicking and screaming, to make it my life's work.

This book is the result of that enquiry, the subsequent research and ongoing practice of releasing trauma; my own and my clients. Whilst its perspective is based on my personal experience and subsequent clinical practice, its theoretical framework is research evidence based as I hope I will show you. These theories, though they may seem unusual, are consistent with science.

I hope in reading it, it becomes a journey for you too where you learn more about yourself, how the mindbody[1] functions and what can be done in a practical way to enhance the body's immense natural capacity for healing. In reading this book and learning what trauma/ unresolved emotion is and how it subtly undermines us, you too might seek to uncover and resolve your past so that you can move forward into your future unencumbered. It is not a self-help manual although you could use it as such if you follow the suggestions and the links to further information. It is not a practitioner manual although practitioners in other fields will find it useful I think. It is a story, first and foremost, about what it means to be human in this point in our history and how we might, in healing ourselves, heal our world. Never has there been a greater need.

Trauma is more common than you think

When you ask most people what trauma is I'm sure they'd come up with the well know stressors of bereavement, divorce, accident, etc. These are indeed traumas to most people who suffer them. They are referred to by psychologists as 'Big-T' traumas. For a long while they were the only ones that were investigated; war trauma was a well-known problem from the First World War (known as 'shell-shock'). But it was not thought of as common, and sufferers were regarded as malingerers or pathologically ill rather than suffering an understandable set of symptoms as the inevitable result of trauma. Then in the 1990's psychologists began to become aware of the depth of trauma from childhood abuse as survivors began to feel free to tell their stories[2]. However, there are other causes that are not so well known even amongst professional therapists.

We have come to understand that "common occurrences can produce traumatic after effects that are just as debilitating as those experienced by veterans of combat or survivors of abuse"[2,3,4]. People can get symptoms of PTSD from these 'everyday' experiences a fact that which is still not recognised by the mental health professional bodies, for example the

---

1 The same as holistic but is more accurate as we now know that mind and body are not separate. Mind is in fact a process of the brain and the brain is an organ of the body.

2 The initial treatment of these traumas was to confront the abuser (who was often in the family) and seek retribution. But the aggression of this approach which often led to denial by the offender, confusion and blame within the family, and subsequent withdrawal of family support from the accuser was often re-traumatising rather than helpful

committee that publishes the psychiatrists' manual, the APA[1] . These are the 'small-t' traumas or Adverse Life Experiences (ACE's) which include birth (especially with forceps or injections into the foetus), surgery (including dental), bullying, anxious or inconsistent parenting, poor parental attachment, betrayal, etc.

These events, which may pass unnoticed by most people, can be *perceived as a threat to the self* by a sensitised child and are coded traumatically in the brain. Quite why this occurs and what the precursors are we are only just beginning to find out. The important thing to note is - *it's common* – in fact one leading psychologist has said that it's "the best kept secret of our culture"[5]. If you doubt this because of the connotations of the word trauma then think of it as unresolved emotional memory; certainly it's pretty much impossible to get through a childhood without some![6] What makes that turn into a pathological process is harder to determine. It seems it is not the event itself, per se, but *the meaning or interpretation* the person makes of that event which turns it into something traumatic - *helplessness* seems to be key as we will see. It occurs in about 20 – 30% of people and is highly affected by the age at which the trauma occurs. Children are particularly susceptible as are women more than men. These early events can then affect the person throughout their life without the gradual fading of normal memories as I will describe.

So, in order to illustrate how these experiences can accumulate even in an ordinary childhood I want to start at the beginning with my story. I have used specific events in my childhood to begin to pick apart how and why these events are perceived by our mindbody as a threat to survival. Please understand that I use my own case not to blame anyone (my parents least of all), but to illustrate how small cumulative experiences, particularly when they relate to feelings of *shame*, can be as traumatic as the big events. I hope that it will be a relevant introduction to what follows in the more scientific chapters. I have highlighted relevant points in italics below specific parts of the story.

---

1 Personal communication from Dr Bessel van der Kolk at a 2015 meeting on Trauma and the body.

PART ONE – Everyday Trauma in a 'normal' childhood

CHAPTER 1 - MY STORY

I'm the product of a 'normal' 1970's childhood (what I now like to think of as 'normally dysfunctional'). I was born in 1964, the second child of an average working class family 'with aspirations'. By that I mean we were encouraged to get a good education in order to avoid the fate of my father who, despite being a highly intelligent man, was denied a university education because of his background (university education for his generation was only for the wealthy). He was a very skilled engineer and eventually launched his own business with a partner and became an 'entrepreneur' but I have to say that didn't really impinge on my memory of him; I didn't see him as someone in control of his life.

[A parental figure can significantly affect how a child perceives the world – a child will learn their boundaries that way. My message was 'the world is dangerous - be careful – you need to be on alert for threat'.]

My Mum must have been anxious when she carried me. The winter of 1964 was a very cold one (like the winter before, the temperature rarely went above freezing – in the UK this is rare). She had had a miscarriage between my brother and me and so I was the longed-for second child – and a girl, finally. My brother tells me my birth was traumatic; I was born with a birthmark because, heavily sedated, she pushed too soon. My mum seems to have blanked this out and can't remember much about it. She's elderly now and said to me 'it's a long time ago' so I guess she has conveniently forgotten.

[Birth trauma is very common and affects both mother and child. The stress hormones circulating in the mother's blood directly transfer to the child who may be born with high stress levels themselves. If they have been subject to a difficult birth also, with forceps or being put in an incubator afterwards then the stress hormones serves to change the way the developing child's brain will mature. There are even some theories that hormone levels in-utero can affect the child's sexuality later in life. Some believe that the child born after a miscarriage has the extra burden of living two lives – that of the lost child as well as their own. The sense of 'never being good enough' is established.]

So, I was the girl to balance the family but sadly I was not at all 'girly'. As a young child, I remember my Mum dressing me up in pink and ribbons in my hair and I routinely tore them out, cut the hair off my dolls instead of combing it and generally acted the complete tomboy. I wanted what my brother had – a train set, Meccano®, freedom! I loved being active, making things and knowing how they worked, I would get lost in books completely, but girly things like dressing up, make-up, etc interested me not one iota. I actually thought girls were mostly stupid, and particularly when they hit puberty and started acting 'all weird' – suddenly wanting to hang out with boys and laugh at all their jokes even when they weren't funny. I was having none of it. I had my good friends who understood me which was enough. I never questioned any of this – it was just 'me'. A few people made remarks and I had some more snide comments to deal with but generally, once in the 6th form amongst the other 'clever' kids, I was accepted. I even had a boyfriend – briefly, I soon realised it wasn't right.

[Feeling 'wrong' or a disappointment in any sense is hard on a child. I have lost count of the times my trauma clients have said this to me; 'I was the wrong gender, temperament, timing, etc'. I have had some clients who reported their parents actually told them 'I wish you'd never been born' or 'you ruined my life'. Such overt cruelty was outside my experience until I heard it in my therapy room. However, more often it seems a mother will manage to communicate this to a child without necessarily meaning to. My Mum never said anything but her disappointment was communicated nonetheless. There was a lack of empathy between us as I felt ashamed that to be 'me' (i.e. authentic) I had to be a disappointment to her.]

My sense impression of my early years was of struggle. I think my Mum tried her best to be a good mother to my brother and me but she was hampered by a difficult childhood of her own (she had been separated from her twin sister shortly after birth and brought up by her grandmother). It is hard to understand now how this could happen but as I understand it her mother couldn't cope and it was thought best to separate the twins. Her relationship with her own mother never recovered and was always fraught. She was highly dyslexic but never diagnosed (it wasn't really acknowledged in the 1940's when she was growing up) so educationally she always struggled and, sad to say, we always laughed at her poor spelling. She worked part-time to be around for us after school but the work was always hard, manual work which took its toll on her.

We might have had a more comfortable life if my father hadn't been handicapped by the burden of paying off a huge debt of his brother's which he took on voluntarily (I didn't know about this till in my 40's – my parents kept this from me to spare me pain I guess). That says a lot about my Dad who was honourable above all else. So he was paying for his own family and the debt of his brother who had defaulted. My Mum had to accept that and couldn't talk about it - it was one of many family secrets. All we knew was that money was tight and it was painstakingly accounted for. I have a memory of Friday nights where my father would bring home his wage packet and different sums of money would be put into different envelopes marked 'Gas' or Telephone', etc. What was left over would be put into 'holiday' or treats such as sweets. There seemed to be a tension around balancing the books.

[*The message of this is: money is scarce and it must be hoarded or it will be wasted. It is also not to be trusted; it can disappear at any time if you get too attached to it. This relationship to money has profoundly affected me too – I find I accumulate money as a safety strategy. For a long time I would not spend it on myself as I felt unworthy of such 'profligacy'*]

Even when I was young I often had difficulty sleeping – either getting to sleep or staying asleep. I think I used to sleepwalk though of course I don't remember this but my Mum tells me that one evening I came downstairs and asked where my brother was and she saw I was actually still asleep and told me to go back to bed. I have a strange recollection also of often getting out of my bed and going to my parents' bedroom where I would climb in between them. This must have been awfully frustrating for them but the solution they came up with was rather strange by modern standards. They decided to fix a lock to my bedroom door – on the outside – it was a bolt I remember. The idea was to deter me but I soon found out a way of shaking the door till the bolt drew across. I don't remember my motivation in doing this other than I hated being locked in. Of course, knowing I was not meant to get into their bed, I would take a sheet and camp outside their room. My mum has no recollection of this now which is odd as I remember it distinctly. I remember being desperate for the comfort of being with them, and my mum's anger when she discovered me outside their bedroom door in the morning.

[*I was clearly showing signs of separation anxiety here. Sleepwalking and night terrors can often be signs of early trauma. The way my parents dealt with the problem would not be considered a good model now but I imagine they were at their wit's end trying to figure out what to do with me.*]

I suffered on and off from non-specific digestive problems throughout my childhood. I was a sensitive child who often suffered 'heatstroke' (headaches and nausea if I got too hot) and abdominal pain. It was put down to a 'grumbling appendix' (what a lovely vague term!). One evening I remember the doctor was called out as it was particularly painful. I was in bed and as he examined me, he was pressing around my pelvic area and he said over me "Mm, you're going to have terrible trouble having children when you're older". It was more a comment to my mother than me (I must have been perhaps 10 or 11 so although I knew where babies came from, I had no clue by what measure he was making such a judgment). I now know that he was referring to my narrow pelvic girdle rather than any particular failure on my part. But of course, at the time that sounded like a terrible prophesy and I believed it was somehow my fault or a failure in me.

[I do believe that my doubt/ conflict about having children was influenced by that comment. After all, this was a doctor saying this which meant it must be true. I was too young to know that he was not referring to me per se but a feature of my anatomy. Of course plenty of women smaller than me successfully have children. It was a very odd thing to say and completely unrelated to my problem at the time. I did not like this doctor, but my mother trusted him and I was powerless to disagree. He did not do much for my digestive problems either which were probably trauma-related. The digestive system is very affected by stress as we will see later].

My brother was 8 years older than me which meant by the time I was old enough to remember him he was out most of the time being a teenager. Our relationship was somewhat difficult. I think he resented me getting all the attention and the age gap meant we never really spent much time together and if we did it would invariably end up in a fight. My memories of him are that he was largely absent or, when he was around, teasing me mercilessly and sometimes physically. His favourite trick was to lift me up by my legs and dangle me over his shoulder laughing as I struggled to be released. He called it the 'fireman's lift'. It terrified and frustrated me to be so helpless. Eventually, I learnt not to fight back as that just made him more determined to win the fight. Instead, I developed the only weapon I had – I was cleverer than him and I worked hard at school to prove it.

[Sibling rivalry leading to bullying or taunting is a huge source of shame which can result in a disrupted adult relationship. Of course a certain amount is normal and just has to be dealt with, however there is a line that can be crossed when a more powerful sibling routinely taunts the other. It is not a trivial thing to be constantly humiliated and for parents to not intervene to prevent this happening. Because of growing up together, a sibling knows only too well how to torment the other, and if not addressed it is something that becomes habitual. My brother says I have a selective memory as he remembers playing soldiers with me quite happily – he's right of course – I have remembered the traumatic component].

My school was a mixed comprehensive (part of the 1970's radical new idea of teaching pupils of all abilities together) but it had only just been converted from a grammar school, was a bit more selective therefore and a lot of my fellow pupils were from more middle-class backgrounds. Their parents were professional; teachers, doctors, public administrators, etc so they naturally were expected to do well and got much support with their school work. I had to work twice as hard to keep up as I had nobody to help me at home. I developed the reputation of an egg-head, which is not very attractive.

I had ginger hair, no two ways about it. Dress it up as 'redhead', 'strawberry blond' or whatever but to my schoolmates and my tormentors 'ginger' was the epithet used. I felt different, that's for sure. I hope it's not the same these days, now that it's more common and there are more of us around. But it set me apart. I was always taunted from my earliest years. There was only one other redhead in the school, a boy who got taunted too but not so badly. I guess being female and ginger just about tops the poll! I was shamed routinely, particularly when, around 11, I started to develop underarm hair. I remember children pointing and laughing, as it too, was ginger. I hastily used depilatory creams to remove it (oh the burning pain of that) but the shame remained. I was 'other' and they weren't about to let me forget it. So, I learned to expect it and my defences, such as they were, were honed. I would be clever and quiet so as not to draw attention to myself unnecessarily. I lived in a twilight world of my friends and my books.

[Bullying, even if it doesn't extend to physical violence, serves to traumatise a child if they are sensitised as I was. A child's personality is formed as a result of these and other life experiences – of course there is some influence of genetics and, as I have said the gestation and birth experience. But there is no doubt that many of the unquestioned beliefs that a child will have are as a result of their early experience and the defenses and habits learned unconsciously from coming up against these.]

Despite the occasional bullying, school was generally my safety valve as I could keep my head down to escape notice but I can remember a particularly traumatic experience when I was about 7 or 8 in my English class. We were learning to write 'longhand' for the first time. I was diligent but I had already started to detect when there was a quicker/better way to do something and I had no truck with routine or established ways of doing things. The teacher had given us all a task to do several lines of 'joined-up 'O's' and I was bored and confident that I could do this easily. I made the fateful decision to do them as a series of loops (rather like a spring) instead of the required flat top of a 'proper' O. I remember queuing up to show my work to our teacher who was a youngish woman who we all knew was frustrated by teaching and not a happy woman. Most of us were scared of her to some extent but I had never had any reason to fear her personally as I was 'clever' so I usually escaped notice.

On this particular day however I was not to be let off so lightly. I showed her my line of squiggles with the immortal words 'will this do?' and she looked astonished and then extremely angry. She seemed to physically explode and exclaimed loudly in front of everyone how lazy and incompetent I was and threw my work with flourish into the bin, exclaiming it was 'only fit for the trash'. We didn't use the word trash routinely then, it was something foreign and American and it somehow accentuated how particularly heinous was my crime. I was humiliated, appalled and shamed. I was told to go back to my desk and do it again. No-one had ever shouted at me like that and I was shaking when I sat down.

[The very fact that I remember this so clearly is an example of how remarkably resilient is traumatic memory. Clearly I know this happened a long time ago, but when I mentally revisit it, it still feels remarkably current. It is something I've never forgotten and therefore is still with me, affecting my underlying beliefs about myself and therefore my behaviour. In research done by shame researcher Brené Brown, 85% of her adult respondents remembered an incident where they were shamed in school such that it permanently affected how they felt about themselves7. As the incidents are usually around a creative act they can inform the beliefs about a child's creative abilities and therefore limit choices in the future. My response to criticism, for instance is not to calmly consider what I could communicate better but an irrational, heart-sinking maelstrom of emotion which usually results in an over-reaction – either a complete capitulation and over-compensation (I'm SO sorry) or, if I perceive the other person as weaker, I may risk going on the attack and try to destroy their argument (the blame game). Unfortunately neither of these methods gets me the desired result. It is profoundly disabling to not be able to deal with criticism constructively. I and many of my clients have lost relationships and jobs as a result.]

When I was 7 or 8 (it's hard to know exactly) I was taken to hospital to have a tonsillectomy (my tonsils removed). I had been suffering from recurring infections throughout my early years (tonsillitis) which were treated with antibiotics which never resolved the problem. In fact they probably destroyed my young immune system and set the stage for allergies but that's another story[1]. It was the era of routine surgery to remove them as a permanent solution (this is not done now thank goodness). It was decided I should have an operation and a date was (presumably) arranged. However, my parents, probably being advised not to worry me, did not tell me this was going to happen until the day of my admittance to hospital. The idea of not preparing in advance is hard to understand now as we would do things very differently. But all I knew was one morning my Mum told me to pack a bag with her as we were going on a trip to stay overnight. I remember I took my teddybear and a nightdress, I can't remember much else. When we got to the hospital the realisation dawned on me that it was only me staying over; my parents were not allowed to stay with me and I

---

1 I was probably highly lactose intolerant, I certainly am now but milk was considered a healthy food then for young children and we were routinely given it at infant school and of course, at home.

was to be left alone – for the first time in my life staying away from home overnight. I do remember crying, and my Mum telling me not to be a baby but to be a good grown-up girl. But she hated leaving me, I could see that and it was very hard for them to walk away and leave me. And I absolutely do remember the terror and loneliness of being alone in that strange bed with all these other children who I neither knew nor cared about running about and screeching.

I don't remember much more about that first night, and the next day went in a blur of ward rounds, pre-surgery medication and then being wheeled into the operating theatre. I wonder if my needle phobia comes from that time as I can't remember it occurring before. The next few hours are a complete blank of course as I was out for several hours. My final memory is of sitting up in bed eating jelly and ice-cream (the only foods a very sore throat can tolerate) afterwards and then playing a game of cops and robbers with the other children. My parents came to visit me the next day and I was home within a couple of days but the experience is etched in my memory as a very traumatising one. The strangeness, the abandonment along with the smell of that ward, is a definite 'felt sense', in me still. When I found out that my adenoids had been removed too (without consent – it was just considered efficient to do them both at the same time) I felt a loss and anger which I can't describe. I didn't even know what adenoids were but it seemed to me that I had had something taken away from me without even my parents' agreement.

[It is well recognised that surgery is traumatising, but there is something particularly about tonsillectomy as it was performed then. Perhaps it was the immobilisation via ether anaesthesia, and the fact that it involves a very deep incision in the head close to the brain but it has been noted by Peter Levine, author of 'Waking the Tiger', a seminal work on trauma, that "many people who had anxiety disorders had also had tonsillectomies as children with ether"8. I still have anxiety around my nose being hit or poked, and nose bleeds are always an issue for me which make me feel very panicky. I wonder if some part of my unconscious mind 'remembers' the operation and the bleeding even though I have no conscious memory of it. I have subsequently read that adenoid removal is a very bloody operation and frequently leaves lasting scars.]

My father worked hard – too hard. He put in such long hours in hot, stifling conditions in that it eventually made him ill. I went to work there in the summer holidays when I hit my early-teens – my memory is of the smell and the heat and tiny metal shards everywhere – on your skin, in your hair and therefore, most likely, in your lungs also. My Dad was ill as far back as I can remember. Of course before I was 6 or 7 he was probably not too bad but I have no memory of that (this is something I now realise is because a child's brain does not form proper memories until sometime around 7 or 8). What I remember is him coming home exhausted, eating the meal my mother had cooked him and then falling asleep in the chair for an hour or so before coming to and watching TV before going to bed. We had very little interaction on weekdays, so it was the weekends where he had some time off and we did things together.

[Another message I subtly received therefore which was to really influence me was that hard work was a necessary part of the struggle of life and it was a noble thing to do to put others before yourself, even to the point of exhaustion. Being sick, ill or putting yourself first was weakness and therefore not to be endorsed. I never saw my Dad take a day off or give in to his illness.]

Illness was just such a regular part of our lives that I took it for granted like people do about their families. As we have no other experience to judge it by we always think that our own home life is 'normal' until shown otherwise. That was certainly the case for me. By the time I was in my teens my Dad was in and out of hospital every six months having treatment for a progressive lung condition which entailed having his lungs drained with a needle (an incredibly painful treatment I now know) and, eventually having one lung removed. I can remember visiting him in hospital after that operation and seeing his despair once the anaesthetic and painkillers had worn off. He said to us 'what's the point' with a despairing look and I can remember my mum and me trying to convince him there was a point in carrying on living – we all needed him.

[So my father had contemplated dying and I was barely 13. My defence was to rally with my Mum and try to be strong for her. In some ways I became her parent. It was a defence to overwhelming helplessness of watching someone whom you love losing a battle with life and not being able to save them. I learnt to fear illness and its terrifying consequences even as it became a 'normal' part of my life. I also learnt not to admit being vulnerable because it caused pain to those who loved you.]

Interestingly when he had had his lung removed he became more disabled so although the regular hospital visits were now reduced (no longer having to endure regular draining) he was very limited in his ability to exert himself and this included play as well as work. I never saw him run any more, or even kick a ball. When we went on holiday the driving exhausted him and he would often have to sleep the rest of the day to recover (my Mum did not drive). I felt cheated by having a Dad who couldn't do what all of my friends took for granted with their parents – effortless play and support – or so I imagined.

He was also subject to unforeseen emergencies. One night his remaining lung developed a hole in it and he was struggling to breathe. My mum called an ambulance and they carried him downstairs on a stretcher. I was asleep in my room. They would have carried him past my door but for some reason I did not wake up. The first I knew of this was when I got up the next morning and my Mum was on the phone to the hospital – unusually as she didn't use the phone much. So, when I opened the bedroom door and saw her I knew something was up. She explained what had happened and that she hadn't wanted to wake me so that I didn't worry. I was shocked – not only that she'd not woken me but that I hadn't been disturbed! I am generally an extremely light sleeper – I wake at the least noise even now. How I managed to sleep through that noise and disruption goodness only knows.

[I wonder if in truth if I was disturbed but some part of my brain kept me from fully waking in order to spare me. Light or disturbed sleep is a legacy of hyperarousal – where the body is on permanent alert it becomes difficult to relax and get refreshing sleep. For many of my clients (and indeed myself in adulthood) sleep is the first thing to go wrong in illness. As a child I would often sleep walk – with no recollection the next day – this is a sure sign of trauma as is bedwetting and/or stuttering. When I suffered depression many years later refreshing sleep became something I craved but could seldom achieve. This is a classic symptom of being over sensitised to traumatic memory.]

When I was 14 there was a shock revelation from my parents. I had grown up with an uncle whom I loved very much who would visit with his wife quite frequently. At that time my parents suddenly told me he wasn't my uncle but my half-brother from my father's first marriage. Both events were completely new to me. I had not known my father was married before; we had never talked about that. My Mum said it was because his first wife died in childbirth and therefore it wasn't a comfortable subject for my Dad. Anyway his son from that marriage had survived and been brought up by his maternal grandparents. It took me a while to come to terms with the fact that my 'uncle' was now, correctly, my half-brother.

My mum was quite clear that this lie had been told to protect me (from what I'm not sure) and that it didn't affect anything really. It was hard for me to come to terms with; for me it was the deceit that I found the most hard. I understood it was not a deliberately hurtful omission of the truth but nevertheless finding out when everyone else knew (my brother knew because he saw some old photographs and, being older, asked who the 'other lady' in the photographs was). It felt like a betrayal. I still find it hard to understand why they didn't tell me, because all the lies that they had to spin around it must have been very complicated. But anyway it gave me a very confused idea of trust. Their idea of protection now seems wrong to me but the times were different to what they are now.

Reasoning with an adult mind, I think the fact that his wife died in childbirth was deeply shameful to my Dad as he felt somehow responsible (for reasons I found out later). Not that he had anything directly to do with her death but it was his brother who was in a Japanese POW camp and had been deliberately infected with tuberculosis. When he was released and sent home he infected both my Dad and his young wife. My Dad got TB but survived (though of course it damaged his lungs so badly that it caused his ongoing illness). His wife though died and my Dad was left with a newborn baby and no wife while in an iron lung in a sanatorium[1] keeping him alive. It's no wonder he was not able to take on the child. I imagine that once their baby was settled with his grandparents (whom he thought of as 'mum and dad') it was probably considered better to leave him there. He never returned to be with my Dad. It's a hard story to hear without feeling so terribly sad for them all. But it was part of the 'mystery' of my Dad's life before meeting my mum and having my brother and me, which he never ever talked about.

[The confusion of these mixed messages meant I never really trusted them to tell me the truth no matter what. I understood that truth has a price and it's often too painful. I wonder if that has influenced me in my adult life in that sometimes I find I avoid saying painful things, even when they're the truth. I avoid confrontation even to this day.]

I experienced a lot of problems with my teeth throughout my childhood which required a lot of corrective dental surgery. Firstly, none of my adult teeth came through straight. I now know that this was due in large part to my high sugar diet (I was quite addicted to sugar!). This not only creates dental decay but it prevents the correct formation of the dental arch which means there isn't enough space in the jaw for all the teeth. A famous dentist in the 1930's, Dr Weston Price, studied this link with diet around the world and found that once native people adopted a Western diet their dental health worsened considerably[9]. But in the 'chemical revolution' of the1970's we had forgotten this important information and nutrition was a largely ignored factor – we were in the era of high-tech medicine where dental surgery rather than prevention was the norm. Particularly as, at that time, dentists in the UK were paid by the number of fillings they performed so it was in their interests to do as many as possible. Dental amalgam was the preferred medium which is unfortunate as the number of fillings I had created many problems for me later.

---

1 An iron lung was the only treatment as there were no antibiotics so options were limited.

['Silver' amalgam fillings as they are still confusingly called, are in fact up to 54% mercury[1] the second most damaging neurotoxin known to man. Still in use and sanctified by the Dental Associations of the US and UK, though banned in some countries[2]. I suspect that their days are numbered. The current official line is that when bound with silver they are benign and cause no more problem than the normal background amount in the environment. However, there is now a lot more research coming to light that shows that the electrochemical nature of the mouth (saliva acts as a conductor) makes the fillings like batteries. This means they then constantly leach low levels of mercury into the tissues of the gums and jaw travelling throughout the nervous system to affect the tissues and organs of the body. Some fillings are worse than others but there is no reliable way of assessing this unless you measure each one with a specially adapted electrical galvanometer. Dental amalgam fillings are highly correlated with thyroid damage and auto-immune conditions[3].]

However, it was not only the number of fillings but the way they were performed that was the issue for me. I was terrified of the dentist. I dreaded them but because I had to go every 6 months for check-ups it was something I could not avoid it. Also, I was phobic about the needles used to administer painkilling injections so by the time I came to have orthodontic treatment in my late teens (too late in fact to save my teeth), I was regularly having full anaesthesia by gas for routine extractions of my overcrowded mouth.

This entailed having a heavy black, plastic gas mask fitted over my face (I know younger readers will wonder why the fuss but the masks were not the lightweight ones we have now – they were more like wartime gasmasks made of a rubberised plastic and they were strapped in place or pushed over your mouth. The gas was then pumped in and you were told to breathe it until you suddenly lost consciousness. I can still remember the acrid smell of that mask. I was often held down at the same time as I sometimes struggled, and one day I remember the dentist said something just as I was going under and one word kept playing over and over in my mind throughout the period of unconsciousness. It was like a nightmare. When I came round there was the taste of blood and a wobbly feeling to my legs – my mum would usually be with me but she would be quick to tell me to 'calm down' if I was a bit hysterical. She was clearly embarrassed by my behaviour.

[Dental surgery is not benign, it is profoundly altering to the physiology of the body as

---

1 http://articles.mercola.com/sites/articles/archive/2013/02/05/mercury-un-treaty-abolishes-amalgam.aspx

2 Mercury amalgam is banned in Norway, Sweden, Denmark, Russia, and largely in Japan.

3 Alison Adams in her book 'Chronic Fatigue and Fibromyalgia' documents the many effects of mercury amalgam fillings and how to detoxify them. See reading list at end.

we now know - the teeth are not dead lumps of dentine and enamel, they have a vascular system which connects with the blood vessels of the jaw. Eastern medicine goes further and describes them as being on the meridians of the body and therefore affecting the energetic balance of the organs. Loss of a tooth therefore, particularly under surgical conditions where they are forcibly extracted before they are diseased (in my case to make way for the remaining teeth in a crowded mouth) is a violent act of alteration to the body. In addition, the utter helplessness of a surgical situation with unfamiliar faces round you, the apparatus of the surgery, lights, white coats and steel instruments are well known traumatic triggers. For me, because this was repeated many, many times in my childhood it became a cumulative burden of trauma which has caused me many issues around having dentistry even in adulthood. Luckily, today it is more possible to enlarge the jaw rather than extracting the teeth so I hope there is an end to this practice in the near future.]

But worst of all I then had to wear braces on my teeth to straighten out the remaining ones. These were metal brackets attached to the teeth and then a large metal frame was worn around the head which would slot into the end brackets of the teeth. I was 17 when I had to wear this and was told I would have to go to school wearing this contraption around my head. I kid you not! I was so ashamed that first day, going into school feeling like an alien. After that first day of being laughed at I utterly refused. I said I would wear it at night, at home. However, the metal mouth brackets meant I couldn't smile or talk without huge embarrassment. Other children had them of course but they were much younger. I seemed to be the only 17 year old on the planet having them and I was very angry about it. Here was another reason to be singled out and laughed at. I tried not to show it but it made me very self-conscious. I went further inside myself to cope, and concentrated on my grades.

By the time I was in my teens then, I was winning awards and regularly coming top of the class – certainly the top girl of my class. I had a rival, a boy who was extremely clever (he eventually went to Oxford I believe), but when I beat him, the few times I did – I was so happy. As I now understand, this intelligence gave me my *significance*[1] and it was to be both my salvation and my downfall in my adult years. I used all my mental resources to achieve success at school and I succeeded – but at a cost to my ability to tolerate failure. I had to have the answer to something; it became part of my persona. My family came to think of me as the 'expert' on everything – sometimes things I hadn't a clue about but would have to come up with a feasible answer. This remains with me to this day.

---

1 One of the 7 needs identified by Anthony Robbins

Sometimes, even now, I have to stop myself from answering a question as if I know the answer. It is a conscious effort on my part. But then, of course, faced with the uncontrollable situation of my father's illness which I could do nothing to help, it was the only recourse I had. I craved certainty1 in an uncertain world.

It was decided, naturally I suppose, that I would go to university; the only person in my extended family to do so. It's hard to imagine now when higher education has been opened up so much that half the population go to university in the UK that, back then, it was closer to 10%. I say this not to boast but to give you the context to my later illness and how these defences that we form early on become a hindrance to us later. I had misgivings about entering university life. I was proud, fiercely so, that I would have the chance to do something that had been denied to my parents (particularly my father – who would have been a keen student I think). But I also feared losing connection with them if I did go. I think I sensed early on that I was 'different', somewhat apart from my family and as much as I loved them, I wondered if going away to study for a degree would permanently separate me from them and the fragile connection I had would disappear.

[I developed a persona that was diligent, and hard-working — to the point of exhaustion – and yet, chronically under-confident. When pushed by others in my class I would deny being clever and would say it was 'only because I worked hard'. I was not given any support in my educational attainment – my parents were unable to share in my success really and my frustration with them was very great. They were unable to help me with homework; I lacked that subtle support for my endeavours as my friends' parents had. They were proud of me but it was a kind of vague belief that I would do ok whatever I did. There was very little guidance (indeed when it came to choosing universities, it was my best friend at school who came with me to visit my top choices, not either of my parents). I had already achieved way beyond what they had. So, I also had a lot of shame around being clever – which is what translated into my doubts about university I believe.]

So, off I went to university – my brother drove me down and dropped me off at the halls of residence. The incredible sense of loneliness when he left was something I'll never forget. Of course, I wasn't close to him so it was difficult to find the words when we came to say goodbye, but I knew something was ending and I wasn't sure what would take its place. I coped with it, as I always had, by being super-efficient and 'getting on with it', not showing my feelings was beginning to be part of my armoury. My first foray into making friends with the other students in my student accommodation was painful. They all seemed so far outside my experience – having the confidence that I lacked and a life I could only dream of. One woman I remember was a white South-African. She was always travelling to and fro. Her bank account became seriously overdrawn in the first term but she laughed it off saying 'Daddy' would sort it out. I couldn't imagine a life so glamorous and unassailable. Most students were from the Home Counties (for non-UK readers that's the counties around London – mostly middle-class and well-off), had siblings at university already and seemed comfortable and confident. There was a seeming chasm between my life/beliefs/ expectations and theirs. I felt like an imposter already. What was I doing here amongst all these super confident people?

[Imposter syndrome is a recognised psychological condition10 particularly common in women – fostered by poor self-esteem and shame. It mostly forms in childhood but develops more significant problems when adult particularly relative to career development where it impedes progress as the underlying beliefs about worthiness are a hindrance.]

Then, one week after I arrived, my world fell apart. My Dad had been admitted to hospital just before I left (again - one of many hospitalisations that were just routine for us as a family). I remember the last time I saw him in the specialist ward he was in at hospital in Middlesex. I was bored. I was 18, about to go off to university and here I was, again, sitting around a bed looking at my poor Dad who looked frail and old (he was only 59 but looked considerably older). It was 1982 and my sights were set elsewhere. I remember wandering off and listening to the hospital radio on a headset near the bed (we had no mobile phones or mp3's in the 1980's). The tune that was playing was 'Save a Prayer' by Duran Duran - somewhat ominous perhaps? When I hear it now I go straight back to that day, and my feeling of ennui but it is tinged with sadness too as it was the last time I would see him. When it came time to say goodbye, he held my hand and looked wordlessly into my eyes. I can't remember what he said but the grip was strong. We were not a huggy, kissy family so there was no chance of that. I knew he was proud of me, I knew he was very sad and in a lot of pain. But I couldn't deal with it so I just felt embarrassment at his obvious emotion, held his hand and said "see you soon Dad" or something of that sort and we parted.

So, when, unexpectedly, my Mum and brother turned up at my halls of residence the first day of term, I instantly knew something terrible had happened. Naturally, my Mum thought it best if I didn't know they were coming. They had rung my personal tutor apparently and he had been able to find out where I was and directed them to the halls. Remember we had no mobile phones so I had no warning. My heart sank as I watched them get out the car and waited for them to arrive at my room.

My first words when I saw them were "is it the worst?" (I couldn't actually say the word 'death') and my half-brother confirmed it was true. And what happened next I remember very well – I flung myself into the arms my sister in law and cried. Note I didn't turn to my Mum for comfort or offer her any support; she must have felt so lonely in that moment. But, as I have described already, we were not physically close and it didn't feel natural to be hugged by her. I realise writing this that it sounds so cruel to her. But there's no point in not telling it like it is. I'm sure some of you reading this will know real human emotions are not always clear-cut like in the movies.

[Bereavement or any form of loss is one of the most intense emotions available to us — it is profoundly life-altering but largely without words. The grief process will vary from person to person but tends to go through various stages; denial, anger, and acceptance — see the work of Elizabeth Kubler-Ross on this1. Along with other emotions, it has been mapped in the brain's system by neuroscientists working on the study of emotions; so called 'affective neuroscience[11]*.]*

University proved to be both my salvation and my ultimate challenge. I had long fought the knowledge that I was probably gay. In 1985, when I turned 21 it was still something to be ashamed of. AIDS was running rife through the gay male community and we had adverts on TV exhorting us to 'be aware' (i.e. be afraid) and 'it could happen to you at any time'. The fact that gay women are actually statistically less likely to get it didn't seem to impinge on public consciousness and, in any case, we were invisible. All I knew was I was 'different'. I had tried having boyfriends but it never seemed right somehow. I never got beyond the friendship part and attraction just never happened for me. What actually instigated my self-discovery was a guy at university asking me out.

We had been friends for a while but all of a sudden he started acting oddly and couldn't be in the same room as me. My best friend at the time was dispatched to find out what on earth was the matter. I was completely perplexed. He told her that he was attracted to me and wanted us to be more than friends but he couldn't tell me. I was flabbergasted. I was very fond of him as a friend and thus was in a complete quandary. I didn't want to hurt him or lose his friendship but the idea of us 'going out' just seemed wrong to me. So, I tried to say as gently as I could that I only wanted to be friends but this hurt his pride and he stopped seeing me altogether. This loss was very deep for me. He reminded me of my Dad physically and I think he had a similar temperament of quiet consideration. In the midst of

---

1 Elizabeth Kubler Ross 'On Death and Dying' describes the several stages of grief

all the testosterone-fuelled antics that characterised student life, he was a rare gem. I had to find a way forward that would rescue our relationship but I was deeply fearful of what I would need to confront. This would mean admitting to myself the 'terrible truth' of my sexuality. I went home that Christmas to mull over what to do. Home was no longer really home to me. My mum was alone now and we did not have a friendship like some people have with their parents; she criticised my taste in food, my clothing and my opinions. I think she found me very challenging – there was no question of 'coming out' to her. I decided I would need to tell my best friend first and see if she dropped me.

It is so hard to convey the depth of shame I felt around this. This was the one thing that my father had deplored, and I had no chance to discuss it with him now as he was dead. I felt I was betraying his memory by admitting to something that was the truth for me. Keeping it private however was no longer an option as my lack of proper relationships was beginning to cause me problems. I had hurt someone I cared about – I knew I needed to be honest but how hard that was, it literally made me shake to think about telling anyone.

[Shame is a big driver of traumatic symptoms and chronic illness. Particularly if you have no support to help you form a different view of yourself. Shame differs from guilt in that it configures as 'I am bad/wrong/terrible' rather than 'I did something bad/wrong/terrible'. It is profoundly disabling and life shattering.]

However, tell her I did and her reaction, thank goodness, was to offer support and to tell me she thought *she* was probably bisexual anyhow. I did manage to tell the guy that fancied me, though it was extremely hard and, although he was disappointed I could see that at least it made sense to him not as a rejection of him personally. He stayed a friend, though when he did eventually meet someone, we slowly drifted apart.

Over the next year I began to build my confidence and experiment by joining various women's groups on campus. I met some other gay women and found that we had a lot in common. Everything made sense at last. I think I was still terribly ashamed but I decided to 'go for it' and at my 21st birthday party 'came out' to myself and my friends. The excitement and terror were equal. I had no idea what it all meant, but I was far away from home and everything seemed possible suddenly. It was a huge relief not to be living a lie. I still didn't tell my Mum. She had to guess, which eventually she did and confronted me. I was mortified.

As is often the case when a person embraces a cultural difference, you can go too far; I was unmissable. I cut my hair short, I wore androgynous clothes, and I got terribly militant about it. I suppose in retrospect, I was trying to make a point, but I suffered badly for it. I was not really resolved, I was just angry. Angry that I should turn out this way when my Dad would not have approved, angry that I disappointed my Mum, *yet again*. I couldn't tell my brothers or take my girlfriends home. I was living a lie of omission most of the time at home and at work. This was the 80's and women often had short hair. People at work generally did not know, I dressed smartly enough and I did not want to tell them. I presumed judgement and rejection which I had had enough of.

Shortly after finding my first job in London I met my first partner and almost instantly 'settled down'. I was still young (23) but I chose someone reliable and capable, I suppose she gave me the first taste of security that I'd had in a long time. We bought a house together; it seemed like a perfect dream. However within a few years cracks began to show. We were not a good match really; she was sporty, I was intellectual. But more importantly than that, she had a fear of being abandoned (as she had been by her parents who sent her to boarding school in England while they continued to live abroad) and I was bored when not stimulated by challenge – I think you could say I was 'addicted to stress'.

[Boarding school or being sent away from home in your childhood is a separation trauma. It takes you away from everything you know, your support structures, familiar places, and homelife. Now, some people blossom in this environment it is true, but for many it is something they never recover from. Recently, the wonderful comedian Robin Williams died after struggling his whole life with addiction. Reading his history it became clear; his early years were ones of abandonment by his mother who was not only physically unavailable as she worked away from home but mentally as she seemed to not like children very much. Compound that sort of early experience with being away from home in a foreign country, as some children are forced to be, you can imagine that their sense of safety and support is lost completely. This feeling continues to affect them throughout life.]

I enrolled on a Masters Degree course 90 miles away that involved living away from home in the week. It should have been straightforward but of course it triggered all sorts of feelings for my partner and my sense of 'having to do the right thing' (people-pleasing personality type) made it extremely difficult for me to cope with. I felt in conflict with my own needs and hers. We survived my year away but at a cost. It was a few years later that I discovered she had been having a series of affairs. I forgave her, we tried to move on but I clearly was not enough for her. My desire to be with her 'no matter what' (I have a tendency towards putting other's needs before my own), meant I debased myself gradually losing any sense of *me*. Eventually she met someone locally whom we both knew and it was clearly over for us. I remember when she made the announcement we were over and I was still in denial about it. You see I could not fathom why, even if someone was unhappy, they would want to break up. I had no model for that in my family (my parents were married for 27 years until my Dad died). It was my Mum's first and only marriage.

I was in a daze of disbelief, a tide of incredulity. I fought it with every ounce of my resourcefulness; persuasion, *niceness* (that's a common one in the chronic fatigue sufferer's armoury), and then downright pleading. It was to no avail. She was clear. Eventually, I moved out and found myself some temporary digs as a lodger in a house nearby. I was absolutely devastated. I had lost everything; my home, my partner and, of course, my identity. I had staked everything on this being the person I grew old with and it had not worked; I considered myself a failure[1]. I was not able to comprehend it really. And, unlike some people whose relationships end, I didn't have my family nearby to support me. I told them of course but because I had never shared the depth of that relationship I could not share what it meant to lose it. They still thought it was a friendship only.

[Lack of social/family support is an absolute precursor to trauma. It even has a new syndrome to devoted to it; 'Complex PTSD' (Post Traumatic Stress Disorder). Not recognised by psychiatrists (yet – it's not in the Psychiatrist's manual), it may nevertheless be recognised soon as more people seem to get it. It is trauma induced by psycho-social factors of failure of attachment – usually cumulative events begun in childhood but continuing throughout adulthood.]

I did what I always do - I worked. Twice as hard as ever. Also, I socialised as much as possible; anything to avoid being in that 'room' – my current living situation was one room effectively. I had the difficulty also of buying out my part of the house when I had no capital investment only a portion of the mortgage that was currently in negative equity. We came to an agreement and I signed away my part of the mortgage. I was truly alone.

Eventually the immediate shock died away and I was doing ok, I even thought I was doing rather well considering everything until about 18 months later I developed a sudden bought of dizziness (vertigo) which was not relieved by rest or by pills. At that time I was commuting to London for 3 days a week (a 150 mile round trip), struggling to make a living as a self-employed garden designer, working long hours but always at the back of my mind was the fear that I would fail like my Dad. Anyway, it was summer and I was doing 12 hour days of physical work and driving but noticing that

---

1 This is shame at its worst. In my world view it was not the relationship that had failed i.e. a joint responsibility, it was me that had failed and therefore was helpless and hopeless.

I felt dizzy almost constantly and my sleep began to be disrupted.

[All classic signs as I now know of adrenal fatigue. Where you have suffered a stressful event which has then not subsided the adrenals are constantly pumping out cortisol until they get exhausted. Adrenals are part of the hormonal stress response and they control, heart rate and blood pressure change and your reaction to infection. I noticed the dizziness most when I changed position i.e. standing from lying down. What I had was 'postural hypotension', a common symptom of adrenal fatigue but neither I nor my GP knew about this; they only recognise severe dysfunction like Addison's Disease. I now know that unresolved emotion from the breakup had exhausted my adrenal capacity to cope.]

Eventually, after soldiering on for another 3 months I began to suffer terrible insomnia which was not easy as I was not in my own home so getting up to make a cup of tea in the middle of the night was not really an option. I would pace around my room, wondering what on earth was happening, fearing I was losing my mind. When the tossing and turning in bed got too much, I went to the doctor and I was diagnosed with depression and put on anti-depressants. This was a diagnosis which I fought with all my might as I considered mental illness was for 'weak' people (I'm embarrassed to say that now but that is the truth as it was then). I was sure there was another explanation.

However, after a year I was so anxious (no doubt lack of restorative sleep was a factor here), that I could no longer kid myself that I was coping. I was put on even stronger anti-depressants. As is normal practice, my GP tried various different pills; firstly amytryptaline to promote sleep (it just made me feel like I'd been coshed on the head) and then Fluoxetine (= Prozac - an SSRI (Selective Serotonin Re-uptake Inhibitor) which made me hallucinate. My GP was surprised when I described I could see auras around people (a light glow) and everything felt very unreal. He reluctantly looked it up in the GP's 'bible the 'British National Formulary' – look out for it on your GP's desk, and found that, yes, 10% of people could have this side-effect. We changed brands and tried something else. I was a walking pharmacy.

During all of this time I attempted to carry on working, albeit part-time. My mornings were a struggle of dragging myself around after no sleep, my afternoons spent 'resting' in bed while I worried that I was going mad. I even said those words to my sister-in-law when she rang to ask me how I was. I remember her reaction was shock but she didn't know what to say so she told me to ring my Mum (not really an option for me really). I guess she didn't know what to say; it's hard when someone you have always known as strong suddenly reveals their weakness. I was still in lodgings which meant I felt I had no control over anything, I was drifting and something had to give.

The final straw was my mad decision to go ahead with a trade show that I had been planning to exhibit at in Newbury. I had a stall for two days and I had to organise purchasing enough plants to make a display in front of me and my garden plans to be printed and displayed on boards behind me. This was an agricultural show which meant the stallholders were mainly land-based companies or selling products to outdoorsy type people. I had to somehow get 200 plants and all the materials into my van and drive to and from Newbury. Luckily, I had asked a friend to help me and she was coming to stay with me that weekend. When she arrived Friday night, I remember she asked me how I was and I couldn't pretend any more. I said 'terrible' and proceeded to cry and asked her to hold me while I sobbed. She was a social worker so knew the right things to say and tried to help me relax but I think she probably was very shocked. On Saturday morning, despite my misgivings we set off and I tried to appear dynamic and interested in all the people that visited my stall. But I felt terrible.

By the Sunday afternoon, I was physically exhausted. I had to go and lie down while my friend ran the stall alone. I was at my rock bottom. I couldn't even muster the energy to drive, my head felt swimmy and my legs had collapsed under me. I was in a sorry state. My friend bundled me into my van and drove me to my Mum's. I remember when she saw me, the shock on her face but she welcomed me in and sat me down. She said 'you're lonely aren't you?' and I recognised the truth of that statement and tears came pouring out. I *was* lonely. I had lost my life, and my purpose, or so it felt. I had struggled so hard to keep going and here I was, in my mid-thirties going back to my Mum because I could no longer make it on my own. I was ashamed and angry with myself.

Over the next few weeks, my Mum nursed me really (thank goodness she was there for me despite our difficulties). She made me meals; she got me out of bed in the morning and generally was there while I tried to accept that I was ill and to cope with the lack of sleep and terrible anxiety. I no longer wanted to go out at all, was quite agoraphobic and I was terrified when she went out – I had to have the radio on to quell the fear of being alone. I was so physically weak I could barely walk – people think depression is all about the mind, but here again, the mindbody link is irrefutable. My muscles ached; I got out of breath even going to the shops and back. But gradually I began to recover my strength. When I was well enough to go home I went for counselling. Another milestone; I thought counselling was admitting you were weak but I was so desperate I knew I had to do something.

During those painful sessions I came to see that the constructs I had created of my life – my 'map of the world' as it is called in NLP, was one of struggle and isolation. I believed giving in was weakness and had found solace in my work, to the point of exhaustion. I realised that living as a lodger was not good for me, the lack of control over my living situation could not continue so I found someone else in a similar situation as me (a guy who had just split up from his wife) and we joined forces and rented a big house together. I hardly knew him, but that first night I slept for 4 hours. The first time in so long that I'd had more than snatches of sleep. I knew then that I was on the road to recovery.

A couple of years later I met someone new and we moved in together. There followed a very happy period in my life where everything seemed exciting again. I think looking back though, that I was repeating my pattern of subsuming myself into my relationship, allowing my partner to be the reason for my happiness and gradually, over a number of years, my unease began to rise again. I quelled it as best I could; this was a good relationship after all. I reasoned that my partner was a lovely person, what could possibly be wrong? But eventually, after a particularly busy Christmas visiting family (and all the inevitable bad eating choices) all my joints (particularly hip and knee) swelled up and even walking became painful for me. I felt very anxious and tired; I went back to the doctors and had blood test after blood test to no avail. They could not find any reason for my pain and I was desperate. Eventually I began to believe nothing could be done (my GP's final suggestion was 3 months' supply of paracetamol!)

In desperation I sought help from a Chinese herbalist – I did not expect it to work at all (a lifelong sceptic and a trained scientist) but had reached the end of the road in conventional medicine. A very kind and knowledgeable Chinese doctor asked me to describe my symptoms and asked to see my tongue (which I had never been asked to do before – this seems incredible to me now – so much is shown on the tongue).

She took a very long and detailed history of all my ailments, took my pulse(s) and temperature and said my body was not detoxifying and they needed to flush out my system with herbs. None of what she said made much sense to my scientific way of thinking but I said to myself, "I'll give it a go – what have I got to lose?" The herbs, as she warned me, were disgusting – the smell of them boiling was quite unpleasant and the taste worse. However, I was determined to try and dutifully swallowed the liquid.

The result was quite dramatic– let's just say my system was flushed out quite successfully!

Then something really surprising happened. Within 3 days I started to feel great improvement and within a week my symptoms had all but vanished! I was absolutely astonished and humbled that my previous opinions had been so wrong. I started to look into this and other alternative therapies – I had some acupuncture to follow up and began to investigate the mind-body connection with reading, learning about other therapies, diet and nutrition. But my partner was not keen, she hated the smell of the herbs, she found my burgeoning interest in all things alternative quite challenging to her way of thinking and I found myself often having to defend my ideas against a person who believed, honestly, that all of this was bunkum.

I think I was split myself – a part of me wanted to explore this and be more open-minded but I was educated as a scientist so I could see her point of view and I felt conflicted often. I think honestly that it was the beginning of the end for us and when we finally parted a few years later I would always remember that the self-conflict was the most damaging contribution to the floundering of that relationship.

[When someone you love does not share your interests that is not necessarily a problem if you can accommodate that within the relationship. However if they mock you and use sarcasm to critique your beliefs you are probably unlikely to make it without great loss to your self-esteem. Partners are often attracted to those with similar wounds but opposite personality styles as it initially makes up the lack in our own personality construct. I think this was true for us but the divisions began to widen as we fell back on our habitual responses.]

Here again loss of the primary relationship was a key element, which served to re-traumatise me with abandonment and loss I had felt earlier with the death of my Dad and the ending of my first relationship. All those emotions came tumbling back as did my depression. Once again I was back on anti-depressants.

[Relational trauma is the term given to such a loss, but it can be any relationship from parental to work, or change of status, etc. The point is the meaning of the loss to you. If you had a lot invested in it and it fails, it can be very significant.]

This time I had some money behind me from the sale of our house so I bought a flat and gradually found my feet again including starting a new relationship. I really believed that this time I would not collapse, but of course nothing in my beliefs or behaviour had really changed. I threw myself into work (by now I had picked up a part-time office job to help keep the mortgage paid) and was managing reasonably well. I do remember though that the anxiety of being solely responsible for the flat was almost intolerable. So many things happened in that flat; I had endless leaks, damp and terrible mould. I feared I would never sell it and move on. I began to realise that this anxiety had always been with me and perhaps what had changed was that my 'mask' had slipped since I'd been ill. I could no longer believe myself to be a strong person, I was prone to depression after all and it could return at any time (this is what we are told).

[Depression is a symptom of unresolved emotion or conflict which triggers the inflammatory stress cycle within the brain and body. It will return if you don't clear the underlying trauma and you are re-triggered. There is nothing to fear if you do the work to clear your trauma or conflict. However it does involve some soul-searching work.]

I eventually moved in with my new partner and rented out my flat but it was a constant source of anxiety and agitation. My tenants were a friend and his girlfriend, it was their first place together and they proved to be quite demanding. I began to think about selling as I wanted a garden and I managed to sort out the damp problem after going through many builders who failed to locate the problem. I sold the flat pretty quickly but not before falling out with my tenant friend who argued about the water bills even though I was on a water meter. I couldn't understand it – why would he think I was lying? He thought it was impossible to have used so much water. We were at stalemate and it hurt a lot that he didn't trust me. We never spoke after that which was a terrible loss to me, but I simply didn't know how to heal it. We have since met and although we have not talked about it directly we have forgiven each other. It was very healing to see how pleased he was to see me after many years.

[I have found attachment to people within relationships to be problematic as my only model was my parents really and I lost my Dad too soon to really be an adult in that relationship. I was estranged from my brother for a long time in my adulthood, we were not close so I had few models for relationships like the ones I was having].

I was beginning to think how I could stay well using all the information I was gathering into my life but hadn't really done much more than that when my sister-in-law (my brother's wife) was diagnosed with bowel cancer at 49. She died within 9 months after enduring chemotherapy and radiotherapy which made her last few months a very painful and frightening time for her, and for those of us who loved her. Once again, I was forced to realise that changes needed to be made – in my life, and those of everyone around me.

[Bereavement again, this time of someone of my generation, was a profound shock. More painful still was the effect on my brother and their children. However, I found it

became the event that drew us together as, for the first time he needed me and I could help him through his complex emotions of anger, sadness and guilt – those left behind often feel guilty for surviving!]

I determined to learn more about cancer – what causes it, how we can prevent it and generally strengthen our immune systems to fight that and other diseases more effectively. The answer, it seemed was largely with nutrition and lifestyle. At that time I had taken a part-time job working in university health research alongside the gardening but I began to have ethical problems with a lot of the studies. Most are based on a model which has been designed around pharmaceutical drugs not nutritional intervention and are largely about making profit for the pharmaceutical industry. I finally made the difficult decision to leave and find something more in keeping with my developing interest in health and wellbeing. I enrolled on the best course I could find in nutrition (there are many out there and all offer something slightly different). I wanted a course that would give me recognition and reward plus the best teaching and awareness of current knowledge. I chose Nutritional Medicine because I wanted to see how food can be used therapeutically. I completed that course at Surrey University in 2008 and, along with clinical massage which I had studied before, decided to launch as a holistic therapist. This would be the work that would allow me to give up the university job and massage/nutrition became the basis of my initial therapy practice.

A couple of years later I went to a talk by a local hypnotherapist at a mindbody group I belonged to. He seemed confident and assured when he talked about various models of mind and how hypnotherapy allowed you to get into the subconscious. I was intrigued. A friend of mine had cured his drinking problem with 3 sessions of hypnotherapy the year before and I wanted to know how that could be done so quickly when he'd had it all his life. This man ran a course locally and I talked to him afterwards, took some details and began a year-long diploma with him in 2012.

I had misgivings and some scepticism I must admit but I was intrigued I found that it was indeed effective, but it wasn't magical or mystical as I feared. It was in fact based on an understanding of depth psychology (psychology with an emphasis on the subconscious programming that we all inherit), and the way it was taught on this course was extensively evidence-based. However, whenever I talked to people about all the amazing things I was finding out about I realised that it has an 'image problem' with the scientific world and with the public. A few people thought I was a bit 'weird' for doing it.

However, at the end of the course, having had myself worked on (one of the side benefits of doing any psychotherapy training), and having completed my case studies, I was convinced this was the missing link in my holistic healing programme and was ready to incorporate this into the next step of my therapy business. I already knew I wanted to specialise in chronic pain. But what happened next was not something I expected; client after client who turned up seemed to have trauma in their history. Hypnotherapy was extremely useful in calming them and giving them control in building their self-esteem but it didn't seem to always clear the deeper areas of belief that were traumatically encoded. I needed another tool in my toolbox. Thankfully that was to come.

Whilst I was engaged on another course (another feature of my personality type is constant studying), this time in healing Chronic Fatigue Syndrome (CFS)[12], I was introduced to a fairly new technique called EMDR[1] by a practicing hypnotherapist, and recoverer from CFS. She was demonstrating this technique to the class and I watched fascinated as she transformed the troubling memories of someone in front of my eyes. The person was clearly transformed from feeling very emotional about something to feeling quite resolved and calm. That happened in one short session; it was so quick. From that moment on I was convinced I had found another tool that was going to be really important. And resolved to learn it.

Chronic Fatigue and Fibromyalgia are sister syndromes with similar symptoms although fatigue is the dominant symptom in the former and muscle pain in the latter. They are complex, multifactorial diseases of gut flora imbalance, hormone and metabolic dysfunction driven by mindbody factors of unresolved or unacceptable emotions and nutritional deficiency. Because they manifest throughout the body, they defy modern medicine's specialty approach, which seeks to divide the body up into different areas of disease and deal with them individually. I was beginning to see more and more people with this condition and I needed to understand it better. I completed my Chrysalis Effect Practitioner training in 2013 and then did follow-on training in EMDR as part of a 'transformation hypnotherapy' protocol. I have since developed this to incorporate other areas of psycho-sensory technique including EFT and havening (detailed in the final section of this book) to create my unique 7 or 12 step Trauma Transformation Programme for people with CFS/ chronic pain/ auto-immune disorders, etc.

These days I gain immense satisfaction from helping people to take back

---

1 Eye movement desensitisation and reprocessing

their power – taking responsibility for their own health and wellbeing by being guided step by step through my bespoke programme of treatments and learning. Each person will be different so their treatment will be different. Just because two people both have problems of 'dis-ease' does not mean that their issues are entirely the same. This is the difference between the holistic (naturopathic) and the conventional (allopathic) approach. You work to regain wholeness, integrity and balance just as I have done (and am still doing – it's a journey not a destination!).

Interestingly the word 'holistic' has the same root as whole and healing. It is however much derided in mainstream thinking. When I originally decided to call myself a holistic therapist another hypnotherapist told me this would prevent me getting any work as most of his clients would think me too 'fluffy'. I have since decided to call it mindbody therapy, not because I dislike the 'holistic' label but because it is misunderstood and, in any case, what I do is far deeper than most holistic therapists will go.

However, I must admit I have not suddenly become 'enlightened' in that I have no more problems. In fact while writing this book I have had to deal with many reminders of triggers of my past; my Mum became ill and has been quite difficult to help as she lives so far away now – there is still a lot of guilt about not living round the corner. I have had some recent dentistry work which has caused my neck muscles to go into spasm very painfully and, finally I am suffering menopausal symptoms of bloating and fibroids which I am trying to deal with nutritionally. It seems to me I'm still on a learning path but am better equipped than I was, so feel a little less overwhelmed. However, I am humble enough to know I don't have all the answers and that each new step I take is important for my own learning. I am currently engaged in doing some work on shame and vulnerability with researcher and lecturer Brené Brown which is very illuminating. I use my experience to inform my work and gain humility rather than for something to blame. I find sharing experience with my clients enables more compassion. However, there is still so much to do…

In the next section I will begin to outline the theories behind what I do in as scientific a way as possible whilst remaining true to my holistic approach. I have highlighted important concepts in bold. Please do persevere, even if you don't understand all the science. I do reiterate many of the key factors several times so you should begin to see how the theory underpins the symptoms of stress and its treatment. It's very important you understand the body is not a machine but an extraordinarily complex web of interconnectivity. We are only just beginning to understand its true complexity.

PART TWO The Science

CHAPTER 2: MIND AND BODY DUALITY

We live in an age when 'biobabble has replaced psychobabble'[13] as the dominant paradigm. In other words everything is reduced to molecules. Depression is simply a chemical imbalance, that with the right chemistry (and of course the right drugs[1]), we can reverse. That human suffering should have any social or spiritual component, or be part of the normal life cycle of joy and pain is no longer considered acceptable. We have a label for almost everything and a 'pill for (almost) every ill'. But still the pain and mental anguish continues to rise – unexplained back pain and depression are two of the biggest causes of ill health in the working population. They are largely treated with the two arms of modern medicine; pharmaceuticals and surgery. Each condition or disease has a specific treatment, regardless of who we are or our life circumstance. Our doctor's time is increasingly limited and there is no consideration of the totality of our experience as human beings i.e. who is the person with the illness. However, there is a small band of people - doctors, therapists, academics and writers - who dare to oppose the mainstream thinking and put forward a more humane view of the human condition where we are not reduced to the sum of our various parts. The reductionist view of modern medicine is failing us in big measure.

This reductionist view has played itself out most clearly in the arena of mental health, a burgeoning problem in the developed world. Mental ill health is rightly considered a pandemic of major proportions and huge cost in terms of lost hours and lost lives. Part of the problem is in our division of mind and body as separate realms; a philosophy developed to keep the church and medicine separate. The philosopher Descartes is generally credited with the idea that the spirit (mind) and body are separate spheres; the mind was part of the spiritual realm which did not follow the laws of nature whereas the body was regarded as a machine and therefore the only part that was a suitable area of study for science. Hence the philosophy of that time (1600's) was that they would leave spiritual matters to the church and western medicine was born[2]. Hence, until just over 150 years ago, we had no scientific study of the mind (psychology) at all. Medicine was (and still is to some extent) only concerned with the body – the mind has its own

---

1 According to Peter Levine author of Waking the Tiger "Drugs may be useful in buying time to help the traumatized individual stabilize. However, when they are used for prolonged periods to suppress the body's own balancing response to stress, they interfere with healing"

2 As Carolyn Spring, writer, researcher on dissociative disorders rightly describes, this was a 'turf deal' with the Pope to keep the power of the church intact.

specialist medical practice - psychiatry.

However, we can no longer accept this old Cartesian[1] dualism of believing the mind and body as separate – both modern neuroscience[14] and the more ancient healing modalities of Eastern philosophy such as Traditional Chinese Medicine (TCM) show us that the distinction is artificial; 'the mind is both relational and embodied'[15]. Terms like 'mindbody' and 'brainmind' are now coming out of the realms of 'new age' thinking and into respected scientific texts. One recent academic author has stated that 'neuroscience is (now) thoroughly monistic'[11] (i.e. brain and mind are consider one and the same with the mind now seen as something that the brain *does* but the two are inseparable from body.

There is a revolution in thinking about to happen. It is based on an understanding of quantum physics. The more we know about how the body works at the level of the cell and subcellular particles, the more we realise how limited was our previous understanding. Quantum biology is a new field that presupposes that in the world of the very small, such as in cells, things behave very differently to the traditional physics of the macro world. Without going into too much detail, atoms behave more as waves (vibrations) than particles. The molecule as the basic unit of biological systems has had its day. This is such a leap that it could almost be said to be a paradigm shift in perspective.

So, the new view of the mindbody is considered much more of a 'dynamic interplay between quantum dynamic systems' rather than simplistic chemical pathways. The pathways we have thus far elucidated turn out to be interconnected in ways that resemble more of a web rather than a simple equation of A+B=C. What we think affects the body in very real (physiological) ways via the medium of the autonomic nervous system (the automatic regulatory system), hormones and certain neurochemicals like endorphins, neurotransmitters and peptides. This system even has a name; the *psycho-neuro-immunological system* (PNI for short) and it finally gives us a mechanism for how the body and mind speak to each other[16.]

How we treat our body affects our mind function in myriad ways e.g. a diet full of processed fats causes inflammation and functional problems throughout the body including cardiovascular efficiency and brain function like cognition. Equally important a life full of repressed emotion or negative self-beliefs affects the body very directly via the gut/nerve axis (neuronal connections from gut to brain) influencing the ways in which your body ages and functions. We can truly call these 'toxic thoughts' and they affect

---

1 The word "Cartesius" is simply the Latin form of the name Descartes

our physiology in ways similar to external toxins by down-regulating repair and increasing breakdown of tissues[17]. Sadly, as we will see, these negative belief systems are all too common (highly linked to shame and other repressed emotions) and are, for the most part, *unconscious* hence difficult to recognise and treat. Trauma is a very *physical* phenomenon and impacts our bodies in very real ways.

The 'gut-brain'

The gut is not just the site of your digestion, as important as that is. It is also a key part of your immune system and the site of a good deal of the information relayed to and from your brain. It has even been called the 'second brain' or *'enteric brain'* as it contains 100 million neurons i.e. more neurons than the spinal cord or peripheral nervous system combined[18]. It is responsible in no small part for how you feel; your mental state, mood and health. For instance, 95% of the feel-good chemical serotonin in your body is found in your gut. This fact has been suggested as the reason why many mental diseases have correlates in the gut e.g. autism and depression often have gut symptoms associated with them.

Finally, via the roughly 100 trillion bacteria that it contains[1], called the gut *microbiome*, it contains enough bacterial DNA to produce a vast array of the metabolic products (vitamins, neurotransmitters, enzymes, and signalling proteins called neuropeptides) that our body needs to function. I often think of the human being as simply a highly evolved, complex host for bacteria! In fact, evolution has shown us that bacteria have often been instrumental to the development of the organism, as they have developed in symbiosis with us[19]. Babies born via Caesarian section often have poor gut function as they have not been properly inoculated with their mother's gut flora via a vaginal birth[20]. This may cause the children to have more allergies and health issues than children born normally, including mental health problems. Given the increasing use of C-section in hospitals, and the likelihood of deficiencies being passed on from that child when she too has baby, this has health implications for us as a society not just as individuals.

While studying my masters degree in Nutritional Medicine a few years ago, what came across to me over and over again was the importance of the gut in general health. Through all the scientific data and complexity that was presented, it seemed the gut was often key. Yet nutrition is mostly ignored

---

1 10 times the amount of cells in your body! The combined gut flora has been called the 'third brain'. Gut and brain start off as the same tissue embryologically. They then differentiate into central and enteric nervous systems. The enteric nerve cells are considered part of the autonomic nervous system in some newer definitions, see polyvagal theory later in the book. Brain, Gut, Microbes; First Second and Third brain.

when you engage with conventional medicine. How often has your doctor asked you about your diet when discussing your mental health – or even your physical health[1]? Now we are beginning to find out just how important the gut and its resident bacteria are. Having a good balance of gut flora may not be something you'd expect to find in a book about trauma and its consequences, but that's what makes this different – I am not looking at purely psychological factors here as I am only too aware that the balance of your gut microbes is crucial to your mental functioning. It certainly was one of the major reasons that I got ill. Unfortunately as your microbes get more out of balance, your digestion becomes poorer, you intake less vital nutrients and your gut gets further depleted and imbalanced. Opportunistic bacteria and resident yeasts begin to take hold. Symptoms are gas, bloating, itchy, flaky skin, cravings for sweet foods, and 'foggy' brain. You can see it is a cycle: poorer digestion – less nutrients and higher yeasts – poorer digestion.

Figure 1 Digestive tract and immunity

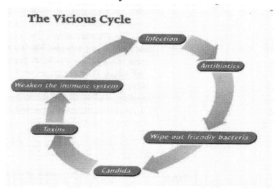

Let's look at one example of how this works. The gut is one of the most important sites of your immune system – the gut wall is, after all, a form of modified skin and as such is an entry point of pathological microbes (i.e. the unfriendly type!). Hence it's not surprising that the most evolutionarily ancient immune function (called the 'innate immune system'), is based here. It is the essential non-specific first-line defence to invasion controlled by the release of inflammatory molecules called *cytokines* –peptides (small proteins) produced in the body which control inflammation. Continuous stimulation by bacterial structural cell wall sugars called lipo-polysaccharides

---

1 While writing this book I had a free GP health check organised by the NHS. The nurse did not physically assess me (apart from to weigh me and take a blood test). She asked a little about my diet and exercise but it was very general and no advice was given to reverse my hormone imbalance.. What an opportunity missed to educate people about health.

activate the immune system to be in a state of constant alert, helping to keep it activated. Bacteria keep us primed!

The release of cytokines is controlled by the balance of these polysaccharides and it helps the body maintain its immunity and, via their or its interaction with the stress response, even its normal sleep pattern (they are involved with the transition to **Rapid Eye Movement** sleep from non-REM sleep). This is important for dreaming and restful sleep. So, the balance of your gut flora influences your immunity and the quality of your sleep; therefore both directly and indirectly affecting your health using bi-products of their metabolism. This leads to the perhaps surprising conclusion that bacteria are essential to our physical wellbeing.

However, they also govern the balance in your mood and anxiety levels via the serotonin and other neurotransmitter levels they produce. Surprisingly most of the serotonin in your body is found in your gut. This is why when we increase levels via anti-depressants (the SSRIs like Prozac reduce re-uptake) you often get gut problems as a side-effect. Too much serotonin is just as much of a problem. So, they are vital for mental health too.

Another factor influenced by your gut bacteria is the permeability of your gut. With a standard western diet (also called the SAD or 'standard American diet' in the US), your 'bad' bacteria are encouraged to overgrow which can cause the cells in your gut to become 'leaky' i.e. the gaps between the cells instead of having 'tight junctions' as normal, develop gaps. If you were unlucky enough to have childhood infections and were then prescribed extensive antibiotics these can affect gut flora for life too and exacerbate the problem.

Bacterial overgrowth can encourage auto-immunity as undigested protein fragments (peptides) and toxins are able to penetrate through the gut wall causing the body to react with an immune response to food as if it were an invader. The cells in the gut are meant to be a semi-permeable barrier, finely controlled so as to only allow certain things in. When this control fails by the cells being permanently open, the barrier is broken and disease may result. Excessive permeability has been implicated in such definitive auto-immune conditions as diverse as coeliac disease, multiple sclerosis and chronic fatigue syndromes.

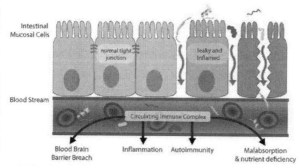

Figure 2 The 'Leaky' Gut

So, leaky gut syndrome is a precursor to many diseases as the gut is key in regulating so many bodily functions. In addition to the direct effects on immunity and inflammation, there are more factors in gut functioning that impinge on your health. The short-chain fatty acids (breakdown products of indigestible carbohydrate in your diet produced by your gut bacteria) are *epigenetic* regulators[1]; that is they help to control what genes are expressed in the cells. These epigenetic effects of the gut flora help to explain why each of us reacts differently to our environment – since each of us has an individual gut flora we have a unique response to the external environment. Those with a healthy gut not only have a healthier immune system but digestion and metabolism work better, with more nutrient availability, more accurate genetic regulation and intercellular communication. It can't be overstated how important this is for brain function, especially in the area of pain response.

Although we are all familiar with the idea of 'gut feelings as a source of information, we are seldom aware how vital the gut is in central nervous system (CNS) function. The enteric (gut) brain really does exist and it is just as important as the brain in your head. Stress (whether conscious and acute, or unconscious and chronic) alters the balance of your gut flora via the release of hormones like adrenaline and cortisol (from the adrenals) and cytokines produced by bacteria. The self-regulating system is sent haywire and the results are *systemic* (i.e. throughout your body). These findings are so important, the study of these interactions now has its own field – Psycho-neuro-immunology (PNI).

---

1 'Above genetics'. It means there is another layer of control above what DNA you have. It is a very exciting development in biology. See the epigenetics section for more information.

Psycho-neuro-immunology (PNI)

The term to describe how the mind and body interact has been termed *psycho-neuro-immunology*. This is a relatively new field which looks at the psycho-social environment (*psycho*) interacting with the mind and body via the nervous system (*neuro*) to affect the immune response of the organism (*immunology*). It's hard to credit that this was ever doubted, but prior to the 1990's this was a rare field barely accepted by the mainstream. Now it has matured into a truly multidisciplinary research area for biological scientists, medical sociologists, health psychologists and clinicians to examine the ways in which 'psychosocial factors such as optimism and social support moderate stress responses'[21].

The most radical part of the theory is the understanding that most of the neuronal impulses flow *to the brain* from the gut (via the **vagus nerve**[1]) and not the other way round. This contradicts our accepted understanding of the nervous system being unidirectional and the brain being the 'director' of the body. It has been shown that the information flow is truly bi-directional; in other words the body sends information directly back to the brain not only by nervous impulses but by immune-modulating neuropeptides which are secreted into the blood stream and return to the brain to give a 'snapshot' of how the body is faring. These chemical signals include the inflammatory cytokines that travel to the brain via blood and via stimulating the vagus nerve where they trigger more inflammatory peptides to be released there[22] (in the **microglia** which are the immune cells of the brain).

As we are now beginning to understand how many common diseases are inflammatory in nature (e.g. heart disease, dementia[2] and arthritis), this has significant implications for people's health and wellbeing. If the gut flora is imbalanced (a condition called *dysbiosis*), the inflammation will just continue to signal. We need to approach both, supporting the microbiome in the gut (with probiotics and reducing inflammatory foods e.g. gluten[3]) and reducing the stress factors (diet, infection, toxicity and mental states)

---

1 The vagus nerve as we will see later is the vital missing link in mindbody interactions.

2 It is even considered now that Alzheimer's Disease may be an auto-immune condition of the brain16 and as such may also be influenced by diet and stress. I would go further and say that most chronic disease is inflammatory in nature and on a spectrum of Auto-Immune Disease (AID). Modern medicine's magic bullet approach might be missing the point missing what is a systemic problem.

3 Gluten is a mindbody poison which promotes gut permeability via increasing production of a protein called zonulin which opens the gaps between gut wall cells allowing undigested proteins and toxins to pass through what should be a selective barrier. The processing and genetic modification has resulted in a form of wheat that has much higher levels of the inflammatory protein components gliadin and glutenin. It has been implicated in anxiety, MS and ADHD.

that upset the gut in the first place via emotional and physical cleansing.

Natural childbirth i.e. vaginal birth and breastfeeding are the ways to inoculate the newborn with a good gut flora (provided the mother is well balanced herself). With the increase in Caesarian births and formula-fed babies these imbalances are perpetuating down the generations. It is no wonder we see an explosion of conditions such as ADHD and anxiety in the young. It is more difficult to rebalance the gut once this has occurred but it is by no means impossible[1] and should be the first line of approach with any systemic disease.

PNI research has led to radical new ideas of the stress function; moving away from a purely fight and flight mechanism to the importance of freeze and the body's withdrawal to conserve energy in times of stress. As Robert Scaer has noted "The tendency to freeze in the face of trauma appears to be a self-fulfilling prophecy, rendering the victim increasingly sensitive to traumatisation with ever-decreasing severity and specificity of threat exposure"[23]. In other words it takes less and less to stress us and the stimulus becomes less specific and more generalised. This could explain the new categorisation of Generalised Anxiety Disorder (don't you just love these terms!) which appeared in the latest edition of the psychiatrist's bible, the DSM[2]. With each new edition of this book, there are more and more new diseases categorised. Is it that new disorders arise from further distress to our mindbody or are we pathologising natural tendencies that we previously overlooked? I'll let you decide your own opinion on that but senior figures in psychiatry believe we are failing people in large measure by our adherence to these pseudo-scientific descriptive 'diganoses'.

Another very exciting area of PNI research is gender difference. Women have been observed to show different stress responses to the male 'fight and flight' mechanism which has been the accepted understanding for over 60 years. One American researcher has called this female effect 'tend and befriend' and says women are driven by oestrogen and oxytocin to nurture and protect themselves and others when under threat. I would agree that from my clinical experience women's response is usually more towards freeze, maybe due to hormonal difference but also women's brains being differently organised as we will see. The freeze response is one we will return to in more detail later.

PNI really shows us that the body (especially the gut) is in constant communication with the mind and vice-versa. We are truly beginning to talk

---

1 Fermented foods such as natural yoghurt, kombucha tea,and sourkraut are often recommended in addition to (or instead of where there is poor digestion) supplements of probiotics if necessary.

2 Diagnostic and Statistical Manual. Contains a list of diagnoses and their treatment.

of a mindbody as a duality. It is an exciting field which holds out hope for a more humane medicine looking at the totality of experience rather than identifying biochemical pathways and thinking that, by altering them chemically we can change function. Evidently we *can* do this, sometimes quite successfully, but the reality is that the side-effects are often worse than the original condition[1]. Side-effects of drugs are the result of having unbalanced a finely tuned web of interactions about which we know not enough. These side effects are not an unfortunate irrelevance but a real cause for concern and, in fact, a *major cause of death* in the US and UK[2].

Epigenetics; genes are not destiny

Another area of recent scientific discovery has been our genetic heritage. When the Human Genome Project was launched in the mid 1990's it was believed that, given the complexity of a human being, there should be upwards of 140,000 genes. It was discovered to be around 26,000! This has been called the 'genome complexity conundrum'. The small size of the human gene pool – compared with the genomes of much simpler organisms' e.g. rice which has more than 40,000[24], was a very surprising finding which baffled scientists. They they could not understand how you could control the many complex processes in the human body with so little of the genetic 'blueprint'. However, they were ignoring the contribution of the bacterial microbes that make up our gut and manufacture many of the necessary proteins for us. They also failed to consider the complexity of the switching system (what turns the genes on and off) which ultimately controls the genetic blueprint.

Before the human genome was fully mapped it was believed, and is still promoted in the popular press, that 'genes are destiny' This is a sort of 21st century fatalism which leaves us powerless and disenfranchised from our own lives, waiting for our inevitable death. If genes control everything and they are a random collection then why bother to worry or do anything proactive – we might as well 'enjoy it while we can' and abuse our bodies in the process.

In fact, as cell biologist Bruce Lipton and others have pointed out, genes are really only the hard disk not the operating system. What causes various

---

1 SSRI anti-depressants are a god example. Touted as the miracle solution to depression in the 1980's and 90's we now know that much of the research evidence was unfairly selected to show benefit when in fact overall most SSRIs are no better than placebo and in some cases worse than making simple lifestyle changes. For some people they induced hallucinations and suicidal thoughts.
2 Death by properly prescribed drugs is the third leading cause of death in the US. See
http://articles.mercola.com/sites/articles/archive/2012/02/11/leading-causes-of-death-cost-for-us-economy.aspx

genes to be read or not are environmental signals that turn genes on or off. This *epigenetic modification* shows us that it is our *environment* (both internal and external) that largely determines what genes are read and therefore what proteins are created[1].

A brief look into a cell shows us that the DNA (Deoxyribonucleic acid - the double helix genetic code) is contained in the nucleus and for a long time it was believed that it was the 'command centre' of the cell, something akin to the brain in the body. However, that was a misunderstanding. As Bruce Lipton has pointed out, if you take the nucleus out of the cell, the cell carries on functioning for quite a while which wouldn't be the case if it needed the genes to regulate activity. It does eventually die but only after it runs out of proteins, which are the actual functional molecules of life. They perform virtually every function inside and outside the cell; from sensing and communication, energy metabolism, structural support, regulation, etc. The DNA code, when translated, is made into proteins so they are considered the fundamental building blocks of life. It is not the blueprint (DNA) but the output (proteins) that are crucial to how an organism functions.

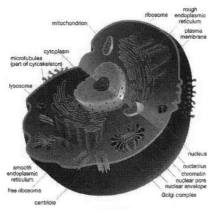

Figure 3 Inside a cell

Equally important to understand though, is that the *reading* of the DNA is also controlled by proteins, as DNA is covered in a protein sleeve of histones which has to be unwound whenever the cell needs to be read

---

1 Examples of conditions which have primarily genetic predisposition are early onset Alzheimers and some cancers. However, they are rare. The more common conditions which affect the elderly are ones that we can influence years before they develop – the middle years are vital.

(DNA is a long molecule so you only read a small fraction of it at a time). There are proteins that not only signal the need for the unwinding but control the process in a highly choreographed way. For example there is a peptide called Brain Derived Neurotrophic Factor (BDNF) that is highly implicated in the stress response. It has been called 'Miracle Grow for the Brain'. It is capable of enhancing the growth of protective proteins, and up-regulating (increasing genetic production of) serotonin receptors for instance. So proteins are the key regulators of life, not DNA.

Proteins are response molecules as well as structural, constantly sampling the environment for clues as to what is needed. These 'clues' may be hormones, toxins, neurotransmitters and peptides, etc. Crucially for our discussion they are also responsive to your thoughts. As we will discuss there are numerous pathways in the body (HPA axis, autonomic nervous system and the gut/brain axis) that communicate not just the external situation but also what is going on inside your body. This 'interoception' (perception of one's interior state) is regarded as one of the most crucial perceptive systems. Gut feelings really are important! If you have negative feelings about something, even if it's not consciously perceived, the autonomic nervous system will respond by sending your body into protection mode instead of growth. As we will see shortly, these systems have been designed over millennia to be protective to your survival and they are very powerful.

If your negative beliefs and feelings are giving your body these messages, the internal milieu of the cell is going to be acidic, destructive (catabolic) and ultimately unhealthy. Effectively your 'filter' on the world is the opposite of rose-tinted spectacles and the DNA that is encoded will be selected by the protein receptors and sensing molecules to be those genes that the body senses are needed for survival; these may be inflammatory and can contribute to illness. The research is very clear; toxic thoughts are as damaging to your body as external toxins[16]. They set in motion a self-destructive stress response.

This process has been described very well by Anita Moorjani in her book, 'Dying to be Me'. She is a British Asian woman who grew up in Hong Kong, so although proficient in 3 languages, she was culturally bound by expectation and found herself living a life that wasn't true to her. Despite living an outwardly healthy life (she was an avid fitness and juicing fan), she now sees that her ultimate 'program' for living was one of fear. Particularly after her father and then her best friend died (of cancer), something she ultimately feared became a reality for her. Shortly after her 38th birthday she was diagnosed with cancer of the lymph system (lymphoma) and 2 years later was admitted to hospital suffering acute organ failure. She was not expected to last more than a few days. She did in fact clinically die for a few minutes, but during that time had a near-death experience (NDE) in which she was reunited with her father and told by him it was not her time. The healing she experienced in her mind when she was able to be forgiven by him, and forgive herself for not being the daughter she thought he wanted was so profound that she returned to her body, to make a miraculous recovery. This is a true story not a fairytale.

Spontaneous remission from Stage IV cancer has been recorded before, although it is rare. What makes this experience so interesting is that it was fully documented in the hospital notes and so no-one can accuse her of lying or of not having cancer in the first place (the usual accusation levelled at such cases). She now makes her living travelling the world talking about the profound truths about living and dying that she learned[25]. One of the things she says is true for her is that the underlying emotion of fear was more important than all the things she did physically and was the definitive reason she got cancer. Now, I know this idea that cancer can be caused by anything emotional is hotly disputed by conventional medicine but it is my observation that emotions do have a part to play (the type of illness you get is often related to the type of emotion you are suppressing)[1]. As we have already seen, there is a potential mechanism via the vagus and stress response, but there is a strong reason that the current medical establishment would discourage this understanding. If people realised that making their emotional health a priority and clearing their negative programming was more important than anything else, then the pharmaceutical approach would no longer be the mainstay of treatment. Vested financial interests are obviously mustered against this, so don't say you heard it from me!

Please understand I am not saying everyone can be like Anita, her experience is obviously a very rare one. We need to be careful not to attach blame to illness as this is counter-productive (it induces stress) but when you begin to take responsibility for where you are in life, you begin to be able to improve your health in profound ways. Remember the control of the expression of your genes is a highly selective process and it is controlled, to a large extent, *by you*. Therefore, prevention is key here. The idea that genes are destiny is outmoded; up to 95% of illnesses are not genetically caused (childhood and some virulent cancers such as that from the BRAC1 gene being important exceptions), it is the quality of our beliefs

---

1 See Louise Hay's groundbreaking book on the subject – 'You Can Heal Your Life'. Equally derided and admired depending on what side of the debate you are on. I have found it clinically useful but am very careful not to 'prescribe' accordingly. It is a guide in my opinion, not a manual.

and therefore our behaviours which ultimately controls the expression. Of course it is important to get exercise and put good food in your body (and in fact I look at this in the final chapter). But people often concentrate on this because it is physical and they neglect the emotional/mental dimension which is more difficult to do. Getting your mental house in order is equally, or probably more important to your health. That is what this book is about ultimately.

Biochemical Individuality; Pharmacogenetics

Pharmacogenetics is the science of individual variations in response to foods, toxins and pharmaceuticals. I have included it here as I think it is an important factor in why we all show biochemical individuality to how we process these chemicals and why some of us are more prone to certain diseases. If you are at all phobic about science and technical terminology please persevere, I will try to make things simple! It is important to understand how this works so you know why we are all so different.

You are biochemically unique – due to your genetic inheritance and your environmental adaptations over your life span. Initially you will have been given a mixture of your parents' genes. Genes are composed of strands of twisted chromosomes composed of the double helix (2-stranded spiral) of DNA covered with proteins called histones.

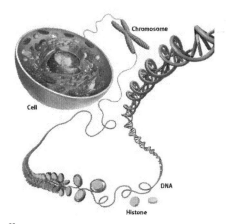

Figure 4 DNA in the cell

DNA is a language[1] of 4 letters made up of paired bases given the

1 In the book The Cosmic Serpent: DNA and the Origins of Knowledge, the author suggests that the immortal first words of the Gospel according to John 'In the beginning was the word' should more correctly be translated as DNA. From the

names A, C, T and G (Adenosine, Cytosine, Guanine and Tyrosine). A gene is a segment of the DNA chain composed of a unique sequence of these letters which are read in groups of three called a **codon**. There are many possible permutations of these codons which form the equivalent of a word. However as we know it is the combination of words which make either an understandable sentence or absolute nonsense. This is what happens in the process of **transcription** from DNA to proteins. Each codon is read by unwinding the DNA and making a mirror copy of it so that it can be transcribed into an **amino acid** (the building blocks of proteins) without damaging the original molecule. The copy is called messenger Ribonucleic acid (mRNA). In computer terms that's like making a pdf (mRNA) of your original document (DNA) to send it to be read while you keep the original untouched.

So for example the codon ACC is a word using the letters (bases) of DNA transcribed into mRNA which codes for one amino acid called tryptophan. See below for a diagram of how the code works as an alphabet for protein manufacture. What is important to understand then is that DNA constitutes the letters, codons are the words, genes are the sentences which translate into the relevant proteins (language) that your body needs to function. But how you *read* the sentences is what determines which proteins are created. Remember that bit if you remember nothing else. There, that's it. Simple isn't it. Here's a diagram to summarise.

---

word logos which means script or language or Divine Reason or creative life-force. Perhaps DNA was around before life forms emerged…I believe we have been given the truth at many times in our history. This is perhaps another dawning of enlightenment.

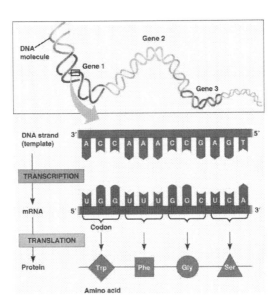

Figure 5 Reading the DNA

Recently it has been discovered that one base (or 'nucleotide') letter may be 'switched' due to errors in the replication and transcription (reading) of the DNA. Such **mutations** as they are called are errors that are generally not allowed to continue as they are damaging to the organism. They are normally fixed as soon as they are detected. However there are certain altered sequences that are allowed, and, in fact, common in the population. These are termed Single Nucleotide Polymorphisms (**SNP** pronounced 'snip') and they will usually substitute one base for another in the sequence. For instance GAC can become GGC in a particular gene 'word'. This means it will affect the sequence of amino acids in the resultant protein *which affects its function hugely*. Without going into too much detail here a protein is not a straight molecule, it is folded and twisted in space like a huge ball of wool. What controls how it is configured three dimensionally is controlled by the different amino acids in the chain. Just one substitution in the protein sequence will alter how it behaves. SNPs alter the sequence.

Over the population then there will be a percentage who have the different versions of these SNPs. For instance there is a gene called ApoE which affects how glucose is handled in the body. It is a very important determinant of your likelihood of developing diabetes. Ethnic variation is noticeable as those from an Afro-Caribbean background will be more likely to have the gene that codes for the less efficient enzyme[1]. **Enzymes** are proteins that enable chemical reactions in the cells to take place much more efficiently. They do this by binding different molecules closer together so that the chemical reactions can happen more quickly with a lower energy requirement. Enzymes are particularly used in the gut where they help to break down food into the constituent parts. They are present in the cells of the stomach, intestines, pancreas and liver. Each part of the gut has a different set of enzymes and a particular function in breaking down fats, proteins or carbohydrates. It is a very carefully orchestrated process.

Liver Detoxification

Liver enzymes are one of the most important in the body as they are responsible for our **detoxification** process; keeping the blood free of toxins, including the by-products of pharmaceutical drug breakdown . The liver is a most under-rated and misunderstood organ. Without it you will quickly die. We tend to ignore the liver because complete failure is a very rare event, and it can function even when it is highly compromised. But liver problems are increasing as we become evermore exposed to the synergistic and cumulative effects of toxic chemicals in the environment. The potential problem with liver function is twofold:

- You will have different inherent efficiency of your detoxification enzymes depending on your genetic endowment of SNPs.
- The liver can be overwhelmed by constant toxicity over your lifespan so that it becomes less efficient over time, but so gradually that you hardly notice or think it part of normal ageing. Brain fog, food sensitivities, headaches, easy bruising and dark rings under the eyes are a good indication that your liver is struggling.

The liver has 2-stage detoxification process called Phase I and Phase II. The Phase I detoxification system, composed mainly of the **cytochrome P450 (CYP)** family of enzymes, constitutes the first enzymatic defence against foreign compounds. Activity of CYP determines your ability to metabolise and break down toxins in the body including foods, toxins produced by your gut bacteria and prescription drugs in a process called **biotransformation**. There are 3 variants of CYP450 depending on what you inherited from your parents. Remember you always have paired strands of DNA so 2 copies of each gene. If both of the genes code for proteins that are deficient, then you are classed a poor metaboliser (this is me I suspect). If only one copy is defective then you are intermediate and if both genes code for working proteins then you are an extensive metaboliser

---

1 Which could explain the higher prevalence in this population

which means you may find no problems with drug or toxin breakdown.

Table 1

Genetic inheritance of CYP gene	Result
2 copies of defective gene	Poor metaboliser
1 defective, 1 ok	Intermediate metaboliser
2 ok	Extensive metaboliser

People in the poor metaboliser group find great difficulty in breaking down drugs sufficiently such that toxic bi-products are left to circulate in the blood for longer. This is what causes the side effects. One class of anti-depressants, for instance, made me hallucinate, which affects about 10% of the population apparently. I was promptly switched to another one. More commonly, though, they will just not work as well if you cannot metabolise them. Nobody mentions this biochemical individuality when you are prescribed drugs, let alone tests for it. You are left to get on with it in a 'trial and error' approach.

Drugs need to be broken down to *activate* them as well as eliminate them so the speed and efficiency of your metabolism has direct effects on the *efficacy* of the drug. If you are taking more than one drug, then there may be combination effects where one inhibits the metabolism of another drug and you will likely get more 'side effects'. This is a considerable problem for some people, usually elderly, who end up on multiple medications. These drugs are never tested together – most pharmaceutical trials are of single drugs in people who have been deliberately selected to *not* have other conditions – so-called 'co-morbidity'. So drug trials are unlikely to find the problems that real people have when they start taking them and in any case the results are cleverly manipulated to be positive[1]. The only way you can find this out is to either get yourself tested for relevant SNPs (still relatively expensive) or trial and error (which seems to be the default position in prescribing in the UK).

Age is another important contributing factor. Most people have fairly efficient enzymes when they are young (depending on their genetic SNP inheritance), but with age they seem to decline. The stomach seems particularly prone to this due to a reduction in hydrochloric acid (HCl) as you age. HCl is needed not only to sterilise the gut contents (important to

---

1 Editors of both The BMJ and The Lancet (repsepected journals of medicine) found that most reported studies are pre-selected to be positive. Since most pharmaceutical studies are sponsored by pharmaceutical companies, they routinely suppress negative studies (i.e ones that show no effect for their drug). There are many other ways in which 'evidence' can be manipulated by a well-funded and supremely experienced pharmaceutical business. See the article by James Davies or Bad Pharma by Ben Goldacre for a fuller critique.

protect you from food bacteria) but to activate the protein digesting enzymes there (e.g.? pepsin). So, people actually become less efficient at digestion with age, meaning more undigested food goes into the intestines to cause problems with the gut flora, leaky gut, and liver detoxification. You can begin to see how all these things link together.

Another factor in your biochemical variability is your gender. Women are more prone to hormone imbalance than men because their hormone balance, being more cyclical in nature and a more delicate balance, is easier to upset. In addition, testosterone protects adrenal function which, as we will see later, is key to the stress response. So, that might explain why more women than men suffer from depression and stress-related disease. Of course, men do suffer from stress, it's just that their bodies (and brains[11]) are wired slightly differently so they will exhibit different symptoms. This is an exciting area of research which is only now beginning to be elucidated. Up to now most medical understanding of the body (excluding sexual reproduction naturally) has been male. Women also have higher pain sensitivity all round, which may explain why they tend to get more chronic pain syndromes.

Finally we cannot exclude the effect your differing history (including your birth experience) will have on your biochemical individuality. For instance, your mother's nutrition/stress levels at time of gestation can permanently change that child's brain development, usually with lifelong effects[1]. We will look in more detail at this in the section on stress but it is worth noting that your experiences and belief systems from childhood will affect your metabolic and hormone function very profoundly, usually for the rest of your life unless you are willing to address them.

Time after time I see in my clinic people who have come to the end of the road with conventional medicine because they have never been given this explanation and have therefore never known what to do to overcome these hidden causes. In the case studies section I detail examples of people who had these unconscious stresses but, with help, were able to reverse them.

---

1 See the work of the late David Barker and subsequent research by the Developmental Origins of Health and Disease at the MRC Cambridge and Southampton.

CHAPTER 3: THE NEUROBIOLOGY OF TRAUMA - THE SURVIVAL RESPONSE

We are at the crossroads of our understanding in neurobiology. As researcher Jaak Panksepp rightly notes, "Neuroscience has enriched our understanding of the adaptive mechanisms that Nature has built into mammalian brains through years of evolutionary experience"[26]. Thanks to the wonders of modern imaging techniques such as functional Magnetic Resonance imaging (fMRI) we are beginning to elucidate the pathways and mechanisms that govern the brain and body's complex interaction via the nervous system.

The Triune Brain.

We are animals – higher up the chain (we think probably at the top), but animals none the less. We have within our brains the vestiges of old reptilian and mammalian structures which still operate when we are under threat. We may like to think that we are logical creatures possessed of consciousness and compassion but, when push comes to shove, we see otherwise. When confronted by something which is perceived as a threat to our survival our thinking brain – the prefrontal cortex (the part that makes us human) is hijacked and the more primitive systems come into play to protect us. Unfortunately, their methods are not well adapted to our 21st century lifestyle of chronic stress and we sometimes end up ill and in pain. We have survived but at a huge cost to our mental, physical and spiritual health.

Figure 6 The brain and evolution – thanks to James Alexander.

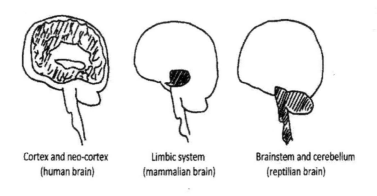

| Cortex and neo-cortex
(human brain) | Limbic system
(mammalian brain) | Brainstem and cerebellum
(reptilian brain) |

The three evolutionary stages and areas of the human brain

You would think perhaps that the brain would have evolved by radically redesigning itself with increasing complexity over time. However, in fact, nature designed it so that we added on a more sophisticated brain over the top of the old one in a series of concentric shells around an ancient reptilian core. This theory of vertebrate brain evolution termed the 'triune brain' was developed by MacLean[27] as far back as 1949 though he refined it somewhat over the next 40 years. It has become an accepted concept today supported by anatomical and developmental studies, although we have begun to see more clearly the interrelationships between the different layers. The importance of this concept for our consideration here is that our reptilian and mammalian brains lie beneath our human one and still take charge when we are under threat. As I describe in more detail later, the readiness to defer to more ancient systems depends on the *degree* of threat we interpret and the *age* at which these events occur. In summary, we have systems that combine hard-wiring from our evolutionary legacy "combined with the imprints of our own personal early experiences"[28]. We are both nature and nurture.

These three levels of the triune brain also correspond to the "three levels of information processing - cognitive (human), emotional (limbic/mammalian), and sensorimotor (brain stem) and can be thought of as roughly correlating with the three levels of brain architecture"[11] So, the functions of the three different layers are:

- basic instinctual actions of the innermost reptilian core of the brain; "primitive emotive processes such as exploration, feeding, aggressive dominance displays, and sexuality"[26]

- the mammalian brain, or **limbic system**, adds emotional complexity especially those related to social behaviour such as separation distress/social bonding, playfulness, and maternal nurturance

- the vast expanses of the largest and final part, the neo-mammalian cortex, to integrate the higher cognitive functions of analysis and reason

There is a functional difference in the three brains in that "higher functions are typically more open, while lower ones are more reflexive, stereotyped, and closed"[11]. What is key in this hierarchically organized system is that the higher level integrative functions of thinking, logic and planning *evolved from* and are *dependent on* the integrity of lower-level structures. So, if your lower functions are frozen and stuck, your cognitive abilities may not be able to make sense of your experience, you may just sense some disquiet, perhaps a 'wrongness' in you that you will incorrectly attribute to being a fixed part of your personality that nothing can change. This couldn't be further from the truth. Just because these feelings have been with you since you can remember doesn't mean they are unalterable. We will see how later.

So what possible advantage could this structural hierarchy have? It may be that this structure of overlaying the human neocortex on top of the older brain structures gives us extra *flexibility* in our capacity to make choices about responding to our environment. Flexibility is what makes humans unique; these close connections from the overlapping human neocortex with the older brain structures enables us to integrate disparate sources of information. As clinician Robert Scaer has hypothesised, it allows us to "attach meaning to both the incoming input and the physical urges (tendencies) that these evoke, and to apply logical thought to calculate the long-term effect of any particular action", (Scaer, 2012). This is what gives us evolutionary advantage over other animals. We can plan ahead and formulate strategies based on past experience using all three layers of our complex brains to analyse, code and execute action.

Meaning, then, is absolutely vital to this information processing as it determines what level of threat an individual will perceive in any given situation and thus which part of the brain will be in charge. It is not the absolute level of trauma which codes traumatic memory formation but the subjective experience i.e. what the person judges to be life-threatening to *them*. This differs from individual to individual. It makes a nonsense of the supposed standard diagnoses of post-traumatic stress disorder (PTSD) as currently defined which can only be diagnosed after incidents "outside the normal realm of experience"[1] like war or abuse. Most people who suffer PTSD symptoms have had no such experience. But their mindbodies still show distinct traumatic pathology.

The study of NLP (neuro-linguistic programming) and now even neuroscience suggests that our reality is a construct based on our 'map of the world[2] which acts as virtual blueprint of our lives. The way we interact with this construct is via connections between our arousal system (the

---

1 Psychiatrist and trauma researcher Dr Bessel van der Kolk gave a very impassion argument against the current definition and being too limited and has suggested a new definition of ' Developmental Trauma Disorder' to cover chronic childhood trauma which is not included in the definition of PTSD in the psychiatrists' manual, the Diagnostic and Statistical Manual or DSM-5.

2 According to Pat Ogden, "we are constantly 'priming' our perceptions, matching the world to what we expect to sense and thus making it what we perceive it to be. This priming function becomes maladaptive for traumatized individuals, who repeatedly notice and take in sensory cues that are reminiscent of past trauma, often failing to notice concomitant sensory cues indicating that current reality is not dangerous" 34. In other words we perceive threat not safety; the bad not the good. It is a selective perception.

reptilian brain) and the interpretive system of the mammalian brain (the limbic system). These neural connections are constantly responding to the world around us compared to sensory input—and these responses consist of our emotions.

Emotions (from the old French word 'emouvoir', to stir up, defined as "a (social) moving, stirring, agitation"[29]) are so named because they organise our need to *do* something i.e. to move in a certain sequence. It has been said that "the brain is an organ of and for movement: the organ that moves the muscles. It does many other things, but all of them are secondary to making our bodies move[30]". According to Colombian neuroscientist Rodolfo Llinas, people experience emotions as the "combinations of sensations and an urge for physical activation" (Llinas, 2001)[31] He distinguishes between emotions and *feelings* which have a cognitive component and are therefore interpretations of our internal emotions.

Sadly for us this system was designed for very different stimuli than the ones we often get in modern life. The feelings people experience today are often such that there is nothing they can actually *do* to express them. There is no movement that will resolve it (or certainly any that we can allow ourselves) and fight and flight may not be an option. In childhood you may be helpless to change what is going on, or you understand that anything you do will make the situation worse. In adulthood, we may repress our natural urges as not being acceptable in our social situation. For instance, anger against our parents, even though very real and debilitating, is seen as unacceptable by our conscious mind. These emotions/ feelings are then driven underneath conscious awareness where they continue to affect us, albeit unconsciously. We may not be aware we have them at all, or we may actively repress them with a variety of means. We get very good at cultivating distractions to feeling or creating rationalisations which seek to explain our behaviour. We are blind to ourselves.

Emotions are thus confusing to many people and when blocked can cause mental health problems such as depression and anxiety as well as physical symptoms like panic attacks and chronic pain. They may interfere with our sleep, relationships and achievement. Emotions are at the heart of what makes us human, the base of both our suffering and our joy. Trauma affects the way in which you organise in relation to the world emotionally. Many traumatised people feel like life is passing them by, their sense of purpose is lost. For some this may result in a numbing to the people around them or conversely they may become hyperaroused to everything and "become limbic" (van der Kolk, 2015). An example would be the speech President Bush made after 9/11; under threat everything and everyone becomes suspicious and the instinct is to attack back.

When emotions are not acknowledged and released, "arousal may drive a traumatized person's emotional and cognitive processing, causing them to escalate, thoughts to spin, and misinterpretation of present environmental cues as those of a past trauma"[32]. The three levels of mind in the triune brain fail to communicate and we are stuck in unconscious arousal. However, people vary considerably in responsiveness to emotional stimuli and thus their degree of arousal. This variation is termed *resilience*, and recent psychological and neuroscience research has been looking at how emotional resilience can be enhanced by what has been referred to as 'positive psychology'[33].

Positive psychology involves a re-training of the brain which encourages people to develop a more constructive, positive interior dialogue by changing the habitual thought forms that we all have. For example by looking at your 'explanatory style' for interpreting your experience (how you explain it to yourself) you can learn to change your experience of life in profound ways. As we will see later in the book, this is the focus of much cognitive behavioural therapy (CBT) and hypnotherapy which aim to help alter people's beliefs about themselves and thus their behaviour (since behaviour is largely driven by your unconscious internal beliefs).

Probably the most significant change you can make in your life is to increase your tolerance of vulnerability – what shame researcher Bren Brown calls 'leaning in'. We so often try to avoid/repress/distract ourselves from feeling anything that these responses become habitual. We no longer engage in any meaningful way with our interior experience – except as a source of fear and reflex action. Instead we create a number of ways in which to drown out the insistent voice of our inner mind with such behaviours as addictions, numbing, perfectionism, negativity and criticism of others. Look at the online world of social media and you will see some of the lengths we will go to deny our own 'shadow side'.

This study of emotional resilience has begun to offer us reasons why certain stimuli which would be ignored by some people are profoundly threatening to others. This is to do with the unconscious nature of much of our processing. Emotional responses occur not by conscious choice but by disposition: limbic brain structures such as the **amygdala** assess incoming sensory stimuli to determine their emotional significance and tag accordingly. This all happens without our conscious awareness. Once the brain has marked a stimulus as threatening in this way, it is *permanently* encoded in the limbic system and brainstem and is ready to colour our behaviour at any moment when the same emotion is triggered. How readily this happens will depend to a large extent on our personality (itself a series of brain adaptations to experience and stress hormones) and environmental triggers. If these experiences happen early in life (e.g *in utero* or the first few years), we will claim it is just our nature, our personality type or predisposition, having never known anything else. Add to this the complication that "traumatized people characteristically lose the capacity to draw upon emotions as guides for (effective) action; emotions can lead to impulsive, ineffective, conflicting, and irrational actions, such as lashing out physically or verbally, or feeling helpless, frozen, and numb"[34]. Arousal is continual and unconscious; a recipe for suffering, for both the traumatised person and those that are involved with them.

Modulation (calming) of this arousal response is possible if early experience allows it; i.e. if a sensitive child has a calm and supportive parent then the likelihood is that the child will moderate its arousal and remain relatively free of trauma. If, however, that same child is brought up in an environment where the parental care is sporadic or unreliable (often the case if the parent has themselves suffered trauma and is emotionally damaged), then the child becomes hyper-aroused and is likely to exhibit problematic behaviour such as explosive anger or ADHD, etc. For some children, the opposite strategy becomes their modus operandi and they withdraw into a world of hypo-arousal. Dissociated from their own overwhelming emotion, they become listless and lacking in spontaneity. These are the children who create a strong internal life which becomes their haven of safety.

Between these two states is the so-called 'window of tolerance' where neither hypo- nor hyper- arousal is too extreme. It is this zone that we aim for in therapy. In many ways we are seeking to make the unconscious conscious, in a controlled and properly boundaried therapeutic relationship. In addition, by allowing someone to witness their own responses from a secondary viewpoint i.e. as an observer, they are able to find new perspectives and develop more appropriate and functional responses. They can both think *and* feel. This is the basis for much trauma therapy as we shall see.

Attunement, Attachment and Arousal

As recent research has discovered, the brain is "hard-wired to connect to other minds, to create images of others' intentional states, affective (emotional) expressions, and bodily states of arousal"[15] via a set of specialised neurons in the brain called **mirror neurons**. They are the basis of empathy and emotional resonance with others. These neurons allow us to interpret the world around us by anticipating the actions of others by studying their facial expressions and bodily movement. Young children will instinctively make eye contact with their mother to communicate, well before they have verbal language. The mother's attunement to this mutual dance of eye and facial expression is absolutely vital in landscaping the infant brain to regulate arousal (i.e. calming the child in the face of distressing stimuli) and thus ensuring empathy between them. If a child is not soothed, and therefore doesn't learn to self-sooth in the childhood years, they are likely to switch between states of hyper- and hypo-arousal at the least stimulus without warning.

Imagine then if the mother is distracted, conflicted, in pain, or depressed. This fine-tuning, which directly drives the neural development of her infant's brain is distorted, fractured and sometimes destroyed. In fact, as the infant brain maturation is based on this "emotional interaction between mother and child, a negative maternal response will elicit a state of shame/withdrawal, characterized by a shift from sympathetic to parasympathetic arousal"[23] producing a typical dissociation or freeze response which many never be recovered. This pattern of shame will result in inadequate development of coping strategies by the child, and contribute to problems with character expression and brain development. Specifically the area of "the right orbitofrontal cortex (OFC), the primary regulator of autonomic stability, may actually be inhibited by excessive elicitation of shame, rendering these infants more vulnerable"[23] to further trauma by relatively innocuous events. Shame becomes the default position for children with this experience.

The future implications for that child, especially if not remediated by the mother or another caregiver later, are lifelong[34]. The child is sensitised to emotional stimuli, finds it difficult to find emotional resonance with others and may withdraw or act out its distress in ways that the parents find hard to deal with. As the child then grows and interacts with other children and adults their inability to self-soothe will create more trauma as their actions are misinterpreted by others and they become further subject to painful experiences of rejection. Many of my clients describe this process of having been misunderstood at home and then bullied at school – a double whammy of emotional pain which keeps them locked into a stress response, their brain failing to break its cycle of fight, flight and freeze.

It's not that most parents are deliberately abusive (although some are); it is often more a systematic failure to connect with their child and create a harmonious living situation (as my experience clearly demonstrates). The child grows up knowing this, but it is a wordless knowing, doubly baffling as no-one talks about it, and in some cases you are given the opposite message 'you don't know how lucky you are', etc. Unbelievably, some very cruel parents *do* tell their children of their disappointment 'I wish I'd never had you', 'you ruined my life', etc but in the main it is an unspoken message of failure. A child is unable to make sense of this duality, and, being a magical thinker, believes they are the cause.

The child then develops strategies to overcome this by desperately trying to please the parent, such as being the 'good one'[1], burying their feelings and sometimes even becoming the parent themselves. They develop certain habitual behavioural patterns that become fixed responses to emotionally charged situations. Thus, if, as an adult they are similarly threatened (e.g. by a bully at work for example), their responses are conditioned by this early experience to those of a child. They will have no idea of this of course, because their thinking brain has constructed a very reasonable, logical argument for why they feel the way they do (rationalisation). For example, the boss is just 'a monster' or the partner in the relationship is 'impossible'. It's the other person's fault because you cannot conceive that you are triggering automatic conditioned responses to similar experiences in your past[2].

Thus, without your conscious awareness, you have contributed to the situation, as you have acted in ways that conform to your map of the world governed by your emotional landscape and it is difficult to perceive otherwise. In subtle ways even your choice of partner may even be dictated by this; often you are attracted to people who have the same experience of trauma but the opposite coping strategy6. For instance a couple I worked with both had difficult relationships with their mothers which left them feeling worthless, but for the man this made him angry and volatile when confronted, and for his partner her approach was to be the 'good one' and acquiesce her needs to please others. They often struggled to be understood within the relationship as each would trigger the other into these stereotyped behaviours. By being able to witness these behaviours rather than get caught up in them, they had a chance to break the old habits and reveal their true selves to each other.

Attachment strategies

Many studies by psychologists from the massively influential James Bowlby in the 1950's through to, more recently, Allan Shore[35], have stressed the importance of the quality of early attachment[3] which directly

---

1 This is known as 'goodism'

2 Eckhart Tolle in his book The Power of Now calls this 'the pain body' which is an apt phrase

influences the maturation of the child's brain for future social and emotional coping capacities. As we will see shortly, it has great overlaps with neurobiology in that we see that social interaction actually down-regulates the stress response[1].

Both interactive regulation (with others) and auto-regulation (ability to self-regulate) are affected by these experiences with our primary childhood caregivers. Most people need a balance of both abilities in order to function well although they may have a preference depending on their psychological makeup and cultural influences. For instance the British 'stiff-upper lip' approach encourages auto-regulation (sometimes unsuccessfully as a generation of boarding school children will attest), whilst the more accepted style of negotiating and talking things through in the US may tip the balance the other way.

Surprisingly, you can observe and characterise distinct attachment strategies even with very young children (i.e those under 1 year old); it is generally considered that there are four different styles (the last one is the most important for our discussion). They are:

1. Secure attachment - the infant shows a clear preference for primary caregiver. Able to self-regulate for short periods.

2. Insecure/ambivalent attachment - the infant anxiously seeks proximity to the caregiver. Attempt to auto-regulate with some help from caregiver but isn't soothed.

3. Insecure/avoidant – clear preference for auto-regulation and may avoid interactive regulation. Often they show more interest in others, books or toys than the caregiver.

4. Disorganised attachment – tends to be associated with trauma and neglect. Difficulties with both interactive and auto-regulation. They may be initially attracted to the caregiver but will then freeze, or be glazed, trance-like, or show other behaviours like squealing, or giggling. This tends to result from an unresolved /ambivalent parenting style. This style can also form through a separation event in the first two years of life – e.g. death of a parent.

Of course most children will not fall so cleanly into one of those

---

3 By attachment we not only mean proximity to the parental figure but also 'access to an attachment figure who is emotionally available and responsive' (see Allan Shore, 2000).

1 For more information on the polyvagal theory in psychology see
http://www.energyschool.com/CSES_Home/Polyvagal.html.

categories, maybe showing signs of 2 or moving between styles depending on circumstance. However, as a general rule we can broadly group children as belonging predominantly in one group. Interestingly, the adult responses of these attachment styles then tend to follow certain patterns also[1]:

Type 1 Autonomous

Securely attached children grow up to demonstrate an 'autonomous style' in adulthood. They make very easy people to work with (so an ideal team leader or head of department). They have an ease in closeness and at the same time an ability to tolerate frustration and disappointment. They are able to accept reassurance and see shades of grey without painful introspection. In therapy they are easy to help as they are able to self-soothe and be helped (but unsurprisingly they make up a tiny fraction of those that seek therapy).

Type 2 Avoidant/insecure.

Avoidant adults are averse to physical contact/eye contact and if/ when they become parents themselves, may not be affected by the child's cries, etc. The child has little emotion in response to this type of parent. Mothers of type 2 are unpredictable, can be warm, affectionate but equally suddenly change and be dismissive causing confusion in the child. As the infant is often hypervigilant to their mother's moods they are consequently less able to explore. As adults they may remain very close to their mothers even though ultimately it gives them less comfort than they need. They are often confused by proximity to others and their adult relationships are characterised by mixed messages of closeness and then shutdown. They may cling or seek to dominate but when their needs aren't met they walk away.

Type 3 Avoidant/dismissive

Children with this type become dismissive as an adult - they are resistant to emotional expression, and attachment of any kind is considered best avoided, indeed considered repulsive by some. There is a strong preference for auto-regulation still. As adults they are confused as to why they are suffering as they have no internal model of their emotional needs. They may also have unrealistic positive portrayals of their families being out of touch with their attachment needs. The thought of being beholden to another often causes more confusion and may result in distancing behaviours. Interestingly they tend to not be comfortable going into therapy and may only come to therapy when something has happened that they can

---

1 For children with any of the final 3 styles they cannot reduce arousal in even moderate stress leading to hyper / hypo arousal in the stress cycle. i.e. difficulties managing stress. Not sure what this sentence means? Few people have a secure attachment so it is not surprising we are seeing a rise in stress-related disease.

no longer cope with e.g. their relationships have fallen apart. They are difficult to interest in internal processing and tend towards intellectualisation. Not a great person to work with in a team situation as they find it very difficult to collaborate. However, there are positive effects that need to be celebrated; they will have been very self-reliant in life and they do well as singles where other types might find themselves yearning for closeness.

Type_4. Disorganised/ Preoccupied

Children of this type may grow up to become frightened or frightening parents. These contrasting styles of caregiving have been well elucidated by Karlen Lyons-Ruth:[36]

Table 2

Frightened	Frightening
back away	loud
quavering voice	intrusive
dazed expression	threatening body postures
startled easily	un-coordinated
withdrawn	mocking, teasing

This is a very common style shown by a non-violent alcoholic parent and results in children who often go on to have abusive relationships or be addicts as adults. We may think that alcoholism or addiction is 'in the genes' but in fact these are learned (conditioned) behaviours consolidated by brain neurochemistry. Mothers of this group have their own histories of attachment failure or trauma, some have PTSD symptoms. When they attempt to go to the crying child they may then get alarmed themselves as they are triggered and so pull away in fear or anger. The result is that you get unresolved parenting – abrupt manifestations of alarm interrupt the caregiving.

Preoccupied attachment results in hyper-arousal problems. Children have a preoccupation with finding someone to help them regulate and adult relationships become intense and enmeshed with poor boundaries. They are often unable to distinguish safety within a relationship and become confused with poor boundaries. We see this particularly with co-dependant relationships which may even become abusive. In this situation they find it difficult to leave the abuser as they have conflated love with control. But more commonly we see that they cannot differentiate between where they end and the other begins. There is very little emotional stability. People with this type of upbringing may have a lifetime hyper-arousal with elevated heart rate, higher cortisol levels with the consequent risks of poor health which that causes.

As adults they show autonomic dysregulation, avoidance, pushing people away, angry devaluing, etc. There are often internal conflicts about distance vs. proximity so they often show a preference for long distance relationships and sometimes affairs (which reflect their internal conflicts with closeness and distance). They may have problems with object / relationship permanence: and fear the loss of someone to the point of actually disabling them. Interestingly this group often become dissociated in adult life – it remains a significant predictor of Dissociative Identity Disorder (an extreme form of dissociation where the person has multiple personalities – formerly called multiple personality syndrome).

Do any of those types sound like you? I can certainly relate to some of those character traits although I may straddle some of the definitions. I am definitely NOT the secure type – I have met those people and you always know them when you meet them. They are quietly confident, sunny people. But they are rare[1].

It's not to say that it's all our parents' fault (after all there is no training in parenting) and that we have no control over this in later life. A good adult relationship can transform a person with a difficult early life and these things are not cast in stone. Clearly we are able to change or I wouldn't be writing this book. But, clearly the earlier and more consistently there was a lack in early life, the more difficult it is to overcome. As therapists, we used to think that the quality of the client/therapist relationship could heal a lot of hurts but for some very highly dissociated people this relationship is the "wrong person at the wrong time"[2]. We are hard-wired to be bonded to our parents or caretakers and when that goes wrong during those crucial early years, it is difficult to undo. Until we have a diagnostic system that recognises that "the consequences of caretaker abuse and neglect are vastly more common and complex than the impact of hurricanes or motor vehicle accidents"[9] we will be missing a huge cause of many medical problems. We cannot treat what we have no language for[3]. Current definitions of disorders such as Attention Deficit Disorder (ADHD) and Borderline Personality Disorder (BPD), etc have many overlaps in symptoms but no systematic attempt at defining the cause. They are designed by a *combination of presenting symptoms alone* and no basis in neuroscience whatsoever.

However, acceptance of where some of our traits come from and

---

1 Some estimate that they are around 10% of the population!

2 Bessel van der Kolk in his talk 'Trauma, Identity and the Recovery of the Self' outlined this theory.

3 At least in the current psychiatric system where a diagnosis is necessary for treatment (and insurance cover in the US).

In the holistic field these definitions are less important. We treat people on the basis of what they present with.

forgiveness (of both ourselves and our parents) are important starting points and absolutely necessary precursors for healing. We all suffer from our own limitations as children. The important thing is to be able to move on from them and clear the residues. Any deficits in identity and self-development can then be at least mitigated if not recalibrated.

Polyvagal theory; evolution and the triune nervous system

A revolutionary new theory in understanding how our internal wiring can affect our behaviour was first identified by Stephen Porges in the early 1990's. He is a psychiatrist who has studied evolutionary biology to develop what he has called Polyvagal theory[1] which overturned the previously held belief about the autonomic nervous system (ANS). This states that there are three levels of the ANS based on the operation of the vagus nerve which innervates all the major organs of the body. Prior to his studies it was believed that the parasympathetic and sympathetic systems were two sides of the finely balanced on /off system. Until then the parasympathetic system was believed to have only one level but we now know that the system is split into the upper (dorsal) and lower (ventral) parts so it is in fact a triune system mirroring the brain's organisation. Have a look at the diagram on the next page.

---

1 "Three neural circuits form a phylogenically ordered response hierarchy that regulates behavioral and physiological adaptation to safe, dangerous and life-threatening environments". Stephen Porges', Polyvagal Theory. Poly = many and Vagal = the vagus nerve or tenth cranial nerve

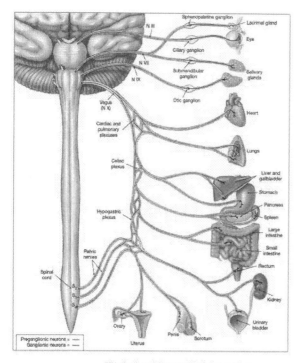

Distribution of Parasympathetic Innervation

Figure 7 The Vagus (10ᵗʰ Cranial) Nerve and related parasympathetic nerves

Note the upper level originates from a different part of the brainstem (nucleus) and innervates primarily the face and head. This most evolutionarily recent part of the ANS, called the **social enagagement system** (ventral vagus) developed to help finely tune the autonomic responses (primarily heart rate) via social attunement between mother and baby. Human babies need to have a much longer maturation before they are able to survive on their own compared to other mammals and our reptilian ancestors. Thus we have developed this sophisticated system to promote maternal protection and social bonding via facial expression, and voice. The social engagement system responds to these incoming signals so that we can finely tune to the subtleties of facial expression and tonality to regulate basic autonomic functions. This extra branch has huge significance for the study of trauma as, being the most recent, it is also the most vulnerable to hijack in times of stress. This idea of hierarchical function was understood at the turn of the 20ᵗʰ century by the 'father of neurology'

Hughlings Jackson. But it is only recently that this third, upper level of control has been discovered and the significance for human development and health has been understood. It has profound implications for human health and wellbeing, particularly in the area of emotional responses to social stimuli which are largely learned behaviours from our early life experiences. If our social engagement system is well developed we know how to interpret others' intentions from their expressions, we are able to control our emotions and develop good relationships with others whilst having well-defined boundaries for ourselves. We know where we end and others begin. This is clearly essential for survival as, if we were not able to bond and be part of a tribe, we would be vulnerable to attack and death.

Figure 8 Nervous system hierarchies

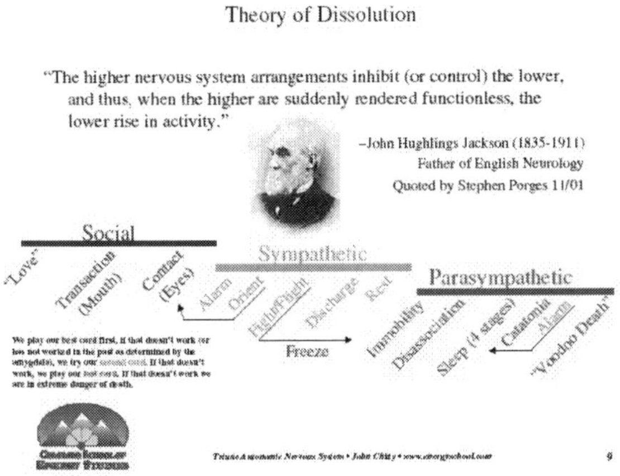

Theory of Dissolution

"The higher nervous system arrangements inhibit (or control) the lower, and thus, when the higher are suddenly rendered functionless, the lower rise in activity."

–John Hughlings Jackson (1835-1911)
Father of English Neurology
Quoted by Stephen Porges 11/01

These three levels of the ANS relate to the era of our evolutionary development they originated in, the speed of nerve impulse conduction and their complexity. For humans in order of complexity we have:

1. The **social engagement system**: formed from the myelinated[1] ventral (smart) vagus belonging to the parasympathetic system responsible for calming us down and giving us time to relax and enjoy interaction with others. Human and primate only. FAST

2. The **sympathetic nervous system** (fight and flight) spinal cord nerves from the basal ganglia of the brain Responsible for allowing us to protect ourselves if under attack. Mammalian. FAST

3. The **parasympathetic system:** formed from the unmyelinated dorsal

---

1 Myelin is the covering or sheath around nerve fibres which makes them insulated and able to transfer nerve impulses very fast so without it the messages are necessarily slower.

vagus nerve which developed 500 million years ago in the fish. SLOW

The important thing to note is that these three systems are *hierarchical*. If the social bonding system (smart vagus) is down-regulated, as it often is with trauma and chronic stress, we will be forced into the level below (i.e. sympathetic dominance) where we are ready to 'fight the tiger'; our heart rate will be high, and our gut unable to function as blood is diverted away from it. Here is why stress makes our stomach churn and our gut is compromised giving IBS symptoms. If our systems are even more exhausted and the stimulus is considered a life threat (as is the case with years of chronic pain or abuse for instance), then these other two levels are hijacked and we operate in the 'freeze' mode of the unmyelinated vagal system whereby nothing works. Our energy levels are so low we can barely function; even the most moderate tasks exhaust us. It down-regulates all. We see this with many trauma related conditions. We are operating at the level of a reptile

For the healthy operation of this 'triune ANS' we need a healthy social engagement system to regulate it. Positive interaction with others inhibits both the sympathetic responses i.e. (arousal) and the dorsal vagal complex (freeze); acting as a sophisticated "braking" mechanism which facilitates the regulation of overall arousal in daily life. When chronic failure of the social engagement system to negotiate safety and protection is experienced, as is often the case in chronic childhood trauma, the system habitually shuts down. Unchecked by the "brakes" of the social engagement system, the sympathetic or the dorsal vagal (parasympathetic) nervous systems remain highly activated, causing arousal to exceed the ability to cope; either above or below what psychologists call the 'window of tolerance', Many traumatized individuals are unable to prevent wide swings of dysregulated arousal, fluctuating between the extreme zones of hyperarousal and hypoarousal"[34].

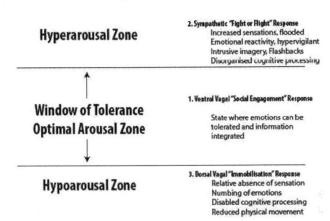

Figure 9 Window of tolerance

The next question is why this social attachment system would fail. It seems that subconscious trauma (perhaps more accurately termed *unresolved emotional memory*) can be the cause. If, in early life, the person suffers a traumatic experience and interprets that they are helpless (and hence feels shame at being so powerless), the memory of that event will be recorded traumatically and unconsciously with the thoughts and beliefs that you had *at the time*. The memories are not properly consolidated (stored in neural networks) so that any subsequent event which bears resemblance to this subconscious belief system will trigger the body to be activated via the ANS, first into fight and flight, and if that then fails, into a primitive survival mode freeze state[1]. The earlier the traumatic event in the person's life, or the more severe the trauma, the more likely this is.

Trauma need not be the major events of our lives; it can be the small terrors, inadequacies and failures. At its heart is powerlessness and learned helplessness, especially from those early parental relationships. You cannot choose your parents (unless you believe that you have on a spiritual level!) so you are forced to accept what you are given. The relationships you have with your parents or primary caregivers are major landscapers of the brain.

---

1 The essence of freeze (dorsal vagal parasympathetic) is powerlessness. Powerlessness has to be present for the body to perceive such a threat as to overwhelm the higher systems.

Their abilities to help soothe you in times of stress are key as to why some children find life very stressful. Freeze response will be more likely when other resources (seeking proximity, closeness and social support) have been exhausted or are not available. This is clearly more likely in childhood, and is the default response then with early traumatic experience. Women also seem to be more biologically prone to this, perhaps due to their relative powerlessness. It seems men are more likely to go into fight and flight, though there are individual variations.

We have certain resources available to us via our individual coping styles, which may involve cutting off emotionally or diversion into intellectual pursuit or creativity but, if these resources prove insufficient in the face of overwhelming or sustained threat, our coping mechanisms are exhausted and we may incur some degree of dissociation or freeze state marked by depression, anxiety, chronic fatigue, self-harming, etc. These can then become habitual responses to stress which the person has no control over and is baffled by as the responses are subconscious.

There may be periods of remission where the person has a reasonable ability to function but as soon as the next event triggers these subconscious beliefs they will go downhill again. Thus it explains the experience of many trauma survivors of periods of relapse and remission. It may even explain the variations in metabolic fatigue common to all fatigue syndromes (ME, CFS, Fibromyalgia), which are essentially failures of the metabolic regulation of the cell[1].

Trauma is recorded as unresolved memories in the emotional brain or limbic system with the sensations and emotions that they first caused. As we will describe in the later chapters, they are processed differently from normal memories and may get here where they continue to dictate behaviour and symptoms of fight, flight and freeze. The implications of this system for the understanding of human behaviour are huge. Particularly in the area of psychotherapy and healing, the polyvagal theory has revolutionised our treatment.. John and Anna Chitty of the Colorado School of Energy Studies have devised a system to support the smart vagus (which they call the 'Social Nervous System') as a priority. Many of their conclusions chime with work that I do:

Health and wellbeing applications of the Polyvagal Theory
    1.   Support the Social Nervous System: With this understanding,

---

1 Trauma is a supremely physical phenomenon, manifesting in insomnia, appetite changes, gut disturbance, etc but psychiatrists are not trained to see this and seldom ask.

the protection and support of the newest and most powerful ANS division, the Social Engagement System, is anatomically and physiologically confirmed as a top priority in health treatments and child care. Emphasize interpersonal rapport.

2. In health care and educational settings, feelings of social warmth will optimize inner autonomic processes for maximum immune system performance, self-healing efficiency and learning capacity (*we could use this a lot more than we do!*)

3. Focus on Betrayal Trauma: Traumas involving betrayal (overwhelmingly painful actions from a trusted person) are known to have particularly deep effect. The Social Nervous System explains these effects. In betrayal PTSD the highest and most modern ANS function (Social) is damaged at a sub-conscious, implicit memory level, with long-lasting, but reversible, effects on wellness and resilience[37].

The importance of this social attachment system is in how it interacts with the various memory systems in the brain. Where we have poor attachment, part of the cortex (the right orbital prefrontal to be exact) goes offline and this shrinks the hippocampus responsible for explicit memory. Memories of trauma are not stored like normal memories. They are stored subconsciously in implicit or 'body memory'. This has very physical effects and may be the biggest threat to your health and wellbeing[1].

---

1 As Carolyn Spring from PODS and many others will testify, recovery from unresolved trauma may be the biggest stumbling block to recovery from the physical and emotional syndromes that result

CHAPTER 4: THE STRESS RESPONSE

The stress response describes the response of animals (including humans) to a stressor which although commonly defined as 'a psychological or physical pressure which is too much to cope with comfortably'[38] has a more biological basis in that it constitutes something that alters homeostasis of the organism. Homeostasis is the internal balance of, for example, temperature, blood pressure, etc is maintained within acceptable limits. It may be either an external stressor e.g. a loud noise or internal e.g. a worrying thought). A mechanism for preparing the animal to fight, flee or freeze depending on what is the most appropriate behaviour, it developed during evolution to allow the survival of the fittest. It is a *hard-wired survival mechanism*, which is why we find it very hard to overcome by 'positive thinking' or other logical means. The stress response is a natural mechanism but it is meant to be short-lived not chronic. A little stress is not a bad thing as it helps us to focus our attention and drives ambition and change. The problem is where it is inescapable, we have no control of the stress levels, and are unaware we are being stressed through unconscious triggers.

Stress leads to a range of systemic physical responses in the brain, the major organs of the body, the immune system and in the stress response system itself. When triggered it activates the **sympathetic nervous system (SNS)** which acts like a police response unit in sending out signals to the body to prepare it for action. It acts in synchrony and balance with the 2 branches of the **parasympathetic system (PNS)** which are more involved in automatic systems like salivation, digestion and elimination as well as social engagement as we have just seen. When triggered by stress this will act like the brake on the SNS so that we are either relaxed and responsive to others or, if overwhelmed, we enter a freeze response. Shown overleaf is a simplified diagram – pleases note it is necessarily simplified as it does not show the detail of the complexity of the parasympathetic chain. But for our purposes at this point it is useful to see it as the balance of two opposing systems:

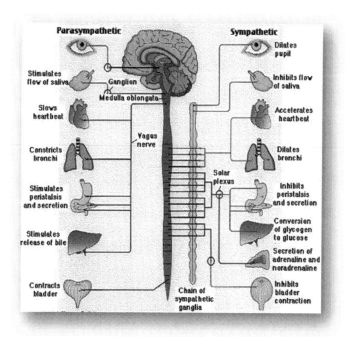

Figure 10 The Autonomic Nervous System

We are only just beginning to understand how the vagus nerve responds to the stress signals in a fully co-ordinated manner. We used to believe that it was either 'on' – i.e. rest and digest or 'off' i.e. fight and flight whereupon the body switched to the sympathetic system so the two acted like the brake and accelerator of your car. However, now that polyvagal theory has shown us the deeper part of the vagus we are more aware of the final level, which comes on-stream when the organism is under sustained threat. This is the freeze response and affects every metabolic process, effectively closing it down. So, with the understanding of the three levels of the autonomic nervous system explained by polyvagal theory under our belts, let's now look at how this modulates the stress response.

Three levels of stress response

When threatened, the mindbody has three levels of response depending on the level of threat. Remember the first level is engaged first and then the subsequent levels are defaulted to if previous levels fail to work:

Table 3 The three levels of response

Social engagement system (Parasympathetic Myelinated Ventral vagus)	Social engagement. Rest and digest, feed and breed	Face, head and jaw including eyes and ears.
Sympathetic system (SNS) (basal ganglia)	Fight and flight. Anger, running away.	Eyes (dilates pupils), Heart, adrenals, kidneys, lungs, liver, stomach, bladder, bowel, etc
Parasympathetic Nervous system (PNS) (Unmyelinated Dorsal vagus)	Bodily shutdown or dissociation.	Same organs of body as SNS but with opposite effect

The latter two states are toxic to our health and 'recovery' from stress-related illness is all about retraining the mind to live 'principally in the green zone[47]. So, with this understanding of stress being a supremely *physical* response, affecting many of the major organs and systems of the body we need to uncover more so we can learn how to undo its effects.

HPA Axis and the workings of the limbic system.

Central to the understanding of how the body reacts to stress is the super-system of the **Hypothalamus - Pituitary - Adrenal system** or **HPA axis**. When our body senses a threat to its survival (in the deepest sense of self) the limbic system (emotional or mammalian brain) is activated. Remember, this is the area that evolved from our mammalian ancestors and is designed to protect us from repeating fearful experiences. Unfortunately in our current modern lifestyles it isn't so well adapted and can actually cause re-traumatisation.

The limbic system is our repository for all of our emotionally-laden memories, sensations and wordless understanding of the world – mostly downloaded when we were young (pre age 7). It is both evolutionarily more primitive and forms earlier in development than the cortex.

Limbic system:

Thalamus - relay station (from all the senses)

Hypothalamus - threat evaluator (is it safe?)

Hippocampus - date stamp and our normal memory processing centre)

Amygdala - fire alarm /smoke detector (& procedural / body memory).

---

47 With thanks to Carolyn Spring of PODS for the idea of the traffic light system and recovery.

When we sense danger via our senses, information is evaluated by both the limbic system and by the left orbital **prefrontal cortex** (**PFC**) (part of the thinking brain) to determine if it is a true or false alarm[39]. The prefrontal cortex can inhibit the amygdala to prevent the alarm going off but if the situation is perceived as dangerous the amygdala signals the hypothalamus via a neurotransmitter called *noradrenaline* (norepinephrine) to send a message to the pituitary gland just below it in the brain. This is the beginning of the sympathetic nervous system (SNS) *'fight or flight'* response via the '**HPA axis**'; hypothalamus, pituitary and adrenals linked together in a coordinated cascade of hormonal and nervous response. The co-ordination of this response is very important in our basic functioning as it protects us from stress and prepares us for action.

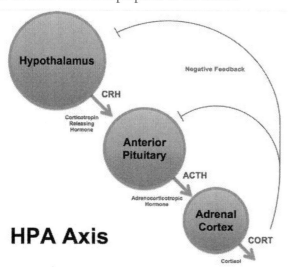

Figure 10 The HPA Axis (Brian M Sweis 2012)
"HPA Axis Diagram (Brian M Sweis 2012)" by BrianMSweis - Own work. Licensed under CC BY-SA 3.0 via Wikimedia Commons -
https://commons.wikimedia.org/wiki/

So, it is the *hypothalamus* in the brain which determines whether the information causes a threat and whether the HPA axis is switched on. If it determines a stress response is necessary it releases **corticotrophic releasing hormone (CRH)** which causes the pituitary to release **adrenocorticotrophic hormone (ACTH)** to stimulate the adrenals to produce various hormones: **adrenaline** (epinephrine), **noradrenaline** (norepinephrine) and, eventually and most damagingly, **cortisol**. At the same time the **HPT axis** (which is similar but involves the thyroid gland) is also stimulated. The thyroid gland in the neck controls our metabolic output and energy consumption. So we have an interconnected response to stress with a cascade of hormones and nerve signals co-ordinated by the hypothalamus which sits at the interface of both endocrine and nervous systems.

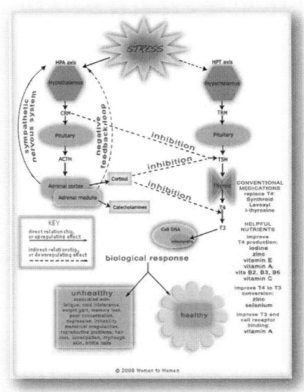

Figure 11 The Stress Response

Note the very important feedback loop of excess cortisol. In a healthy individual excess cortisol will exert an inhibition of the hypothalamus to prevent CRH production which stops the cascade thereby regulating overproduction once the threat has passed. The HPA axis is meant to be a *short-term response* as it floods the body with adrenaline and other catecholamines (hormones with a similar ring structure). These have various effects related to mobilising the body; an increase in heart rate and respiration, maximising oxygen flow to muscle tissue and 'turning off' other non-essential organ systems, including the frontal cortex (our thinking brains). We are in "survival mode," ready to fight the sabre-toothed tiger or run. This worked well for us when we lived the kinds of lives where stress was intermittent and short-term. It works rather badly now that our lives are filled with chronic stress, some of which is unconscious and programmed into us from an early age.

As we are mobilising to flee or fight, the adrenal glands initiate reciprocal activity in the parasympathetic nervous system, the other half of this finely-balanced response unit which is preparing us for the cessation of danger and recovery. A hormone called **cortisol** is released from the adrenals (but a different part to adrenaline; the cortex – hence the name). Cortisol's primary function is to help us recover from stress by metabolising energy – it presupposes action. When the system is in balance these systems work in a complementary fashion to keep the body working optimally. However, unfortunately this is not always the case and sympathetic over-arousal as a result of sustained threat may keep the body on high alert almost permanently. This has several effects;

1. Physiology

In order to prepare the body for fight or flight several physiological systems are activated by the release of adrenaline, noradrenaline and cortisol from the adrenals;

- The heart begins to beat faster to pump blood around the body
- Blood is diverted from the gut (reducing digestive ability) to more immediately important areas like the muscles by constriction/relaxation of blood vessels in specific parts of the body
- Glucose is released from the liver for acting as a nutrient for muscular action and brain activity
- The pupils dilate to allow more acute vision

In a particularly stressful situation there may also be loss of hearing and peripheral vision, shaking (an important way of dissipating stored energy) and loss of bladder and bowel control. These are usually short-term effects. Mainly cortisol opposes the action of insulin to release glucose from cells to increase blood sugar. However chronically high levels can cause many detrimental effects like weight gain, breaking down muscle mass and eventually causing insulin resistance as more and more insulin must be pumped out to counter it.

Cortisol has an inhibitory effect on the thyroid too so you will find that energy production in the cells (within the mitochondria to be exact) also slows down giving us a lower metabolic rate so we burn less. This is the basis of the freeze response. Via a massive release of endorphins ('natural heroin'), we alter perception of pain and slow down non-essential tasks in order to conserve energy. If the body perceives we can't escape then it prepares the body for shutdown. The heart and brain are particularly affected as they use the most energy.

Longer term effects of continual stress are more difficult to pinpoint but for instance may contribute to heart and cardiovascular disease, the biggest cause of death in the Western world. It seems that the effect of cortisol is to constrict the blood vessel diameter so making the heart have to pump harder (ischaemic heart disease means a restriction in blood supply). It may also depress the immune system opening you up to disease such as cancer (which is a systemic failure of the immune system to control overgrowth of damaged cells). Carolyn Spring has said that "excess cortisol from chronic stress is one of the main factors influencing physical health" including the development of diabetes, cancer, etc[48]. Certainly excess cortisol causes wait gain around the abdomen, particularly the more dangerous visceral fat (fat around the middle)[43], sometimes known as 'trauma tummy'. This is not good news; visceral fat has many health risks, unlike peripheral fat in the skin[40].

2. Psychology

The other effect of stimulation of the stress response is psychological. We are immediately set into a state of alert whereby everything we sense in our environment we perceive as a *threat to our survival*. The normal rational mind is bypassed and we move into 'attack mode'. We subconsciously interpret every interaction in the light of this belief and therefore see everyone and everything as an enemy, expecting the worst, looking out for danger even though we may be perfectly safe. It is the perception that is distorted and it will make us overreact to the slightest stimulus whether verbal (a comment) or physical (light, sound or touch)[49]. It is as if a filter is applied to every experience and "fear becomes the lens through which we see the world".[44]

This is unfortunately all too common in our modern hectic lifestyles where stress, instead of being acute, short term and occasional becomes chronic; constant low-level stress which the body has no chance to dissipate. Our ability to negotiate our way optimally in the world and the

48 Carolyn Spring is a director of PODS ; Positive Outcomes for Dissociative Survivors – a group dedicated to empowering trauma survivors through recovery. See www.pods-online.org.uk
49 people with Chronic Fatigue and other stress-related diseases often become hypersensitive to sound and light

way we interact with others is affected and hence our relationships and mental health suffer considerably. We may even become ill with anxiety and depression as we struggle to deal with our internal conflicts; and make poor decisions which exacerbate the problem. Conflicts, as we shall see later, are often registered on a biological level subconsciously and then affect us in successive layers from surface to internal[50]. We enter a downward cycle of dysfunction with the end result that we become overwhelmed and burnout is inevitable.

In a 'normal' course of events (transient threat) we can recalibrate after the event by crying, shaking and trembling so that our cortisol levels go down and our hippocampus can operate to put things into perspective and prepare us to file the memories away properly during REM sleep. However, if the threat is ongoing (chronic), the person doing the threatening is the very person we expect to protect us (our parents for instance), or we have already had previous trauma in our childhood which has sensitised us, cortisol levels remain high. This high blood cortisol level damages the hippocampus and we are unable to store the memory properly and make sense of what has happened to us. Thus we are traumatized and the memory is stored permanently 'in the now' within the amygdala and other brain regions as an implicit (or sensory) memory *without words*. As hippocampal damage inhibits memory storage generally, we also may exhibit memory loss (amnesia) for the initiating event, which has interesting implications for treatment as the person may be completely unaware of what happened to make them feel the way they do[51].

The threat feels *permanent*, and in the *present* – it never decays and is ready to be re-triggered whenever we have a similar emotion or are threatened again. What is also interesting is that the threat does not have to be *real* – it can be a subconscious association with a previous perceived threat (the way a person spoke to you for instance). It can be a sensory learned (conditioned) response e.g. a man with a beard, or the sound of a ticking clock – all of the sensory experiences that were concurrent with the initial traumatizing event are stored as associated memories and they become linked in the limbic system to be replayed when a new threat is present. This is the essential problem of why we feel suddenly overwhelmed but have no idea why; the memories are cumulative but wordless with no

---

50 Dr Ryke Hamer describes this conflict as completely unconscious and biological in origin due to the various layers of brain development and mapping to specific parts of the body in his New Medicine'

51 Carolyn Spring in her book 'Recovery is My Best Revenge' talks of having complete amnesia for her childhood abuse until her mid-30's. This is not uncommon. The mind has dissociated to prevent eruption of bad memories from becoming conscious

narrative with which to make sense of our feelings and we are conditioned to react.

This is the basis of much of our dysfunctional behaviour (fear, anxiety, addictions, repetitive behaviour, etc) and, in my opinion, much of our problem with social interaction. We feel bruised by criticism that may not have been meant, we perceive threat where there is none, and we are plagued by a sense of not belonging ('imposter syndrome). In addition my theory is that it is also a major cause of physical pains that never seem to have a clear cause. If the threat feelings go on for long enough, we will revert to a freeze response but completely unconsciously. We are stuck in a downward spiral as symptoms of illness then add a further burden of stress (being ill is a stress in itself). No wonder we suffer!

Subconscious Stress and its consequences

So, in this book I am talking about stress in a very particular way that differs from the mainstream understanding. We all know that too much stress is bad for us and most of us can identify obvious stressors in our lives e.g. our work, our relationships, money, etc. But less obvious are the subconscious stressors of unresolved emotion, unhealthy beliefs and traumatic body memory, usually from childhood. Because these are held subconsciously in the limbic system which is a more primitive, unconscious part of our brain (and also stored in? our body which reads this part of our mind), we are simply not aware that we have them let alone that they consistently undermine our best efforts to lead a healthy and joyful life.

In a person who has been subject to trauma, the 'stress' to which they are subjected is largely internal, through kindled' (retriggered) memory systems that are activated by spontaneous recycled memories as well as increasingly nonspecific external stress-linked cues. Since these types of stressors cannot be fought or escaped, the inevitable response is a cyclical and increasingly recurrent freeze, or **hypoarousal** (a form of dissociative response) with periodic cycling into **hyperarousal**. There is evidence that the HPA axis in **Post-traumatic Stress Disorder (PTSD)** may be more sensitive / over-responsive to internal biological stimuli. This may reflect neurophysiological sensitisation and 'kindling' phenomena also attributed to trauma. **Kindling**[52] occurs because the pathways become more easily stimulated the more they are triggered. It is the basic reason why trauma gets stuck in the system. What you are responding to are unprocessed memories of trauma, not the current event itself, although it feels like it. As a result you are failing to moderate arousal to keep within the 'window of

---

52 A wonderful term taken from kindling wood which is used to start a fire. It is the tendency of neural pathways of the brain to react to repeated stimulation by lowering response thresholds and therefore becoming more easily stimulated.

tolerance' which becomes narrower as you avoid more of the things that trigger you. You become over-sensitised to environmental signals that remind you of old events. Hence "people are at risk of getting "stuck" in familiar, yet unhealthy emotional and behavioural patterns and living their lives through the automatic filters of past familiar or traumatic experience"[41]. We need to break free of these automatic cycles and get back into our own window of tolerance where we stop feeling overwhelmed and regain control of our lives.

Figure 12. The Nervous System and Stress

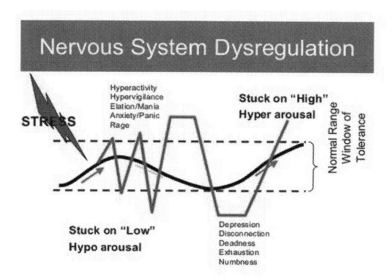

So in this working model, hyperarousal corresponds to sympathetic stimulation (fight and flight), hypoarousal to dorsal parasympathetic (freeze) and the area in between (the 'window of tolerance'), the (ventral) parasympathetic otherwise known as the social engagement system - this is the one we want to keep functioning to enable us to 'rest and digest'. However when subject to stress we tend to bounce around between the upper or lower states of hyper or hypo-arousal. A cyclical or 'oscillating' dominance of these two states has been documented in many disease states: OCD, bipolar disorder for instance.[53] "Oscillation', indeed may well

---

53 Interestingly PTSD (and therefore by extension, a less acute trauma state) is not considered to be a cyclical disease. This is possibly because most of the measurements have been of sympathetic arousal (blood pressure/ heart-rate and electrodermal responses) and thus the parasympathetic effects have not been noted. It is a common experience that

represent a general principle of biological functioning. A system, such as the autonomic nervous system, sensitized by exposure to stressors *without physiological resolution of the resulting response*, will be driven to reverberate, or oscillate, within the limits of its physiological boundaries. This may well be an innate biological reflex designed to re-establish homeostasis"[23]. It may explain certain of the symptoms of hyperarousal such as the 'flare-ups' common in chronic pain, or common symptoms of insomnia, anxiety and emotional instability in traumatised individuals.

It's important to note that trauma is subjective; a traumatic event doesn't always lead to psychological trauma – it really depends on the person's brain and how it has been landscaped or kindled by early experience. Childhood events are always more powerful landscapers of the brain – a child is very vulnerable, not having developed sufficient power or awareness of their environment to either escape or find an alternative explanation of the event other than that they are at fault, wrong or deserved whatever happened. Remember, the necessary factors that have to be in place are *helplessness/powerlessness, fear and a perceived threat to survival*. This is unfortunately a common occurrence in childhood, when a child has already been sensitised by birth or other trauma.

Most importantly then, it is the *meaning* of the stress as interpreted by the brain that modulates the stress response more than the explicit nature of the stress itself. It is the brain's interpretation of the threat that drives the stress response. This has been demonstrated in HIV-positive men, cancer survivors and many other groups. If the person is able to maintain a positive outlook which is not driven by a negative belief system, they are less likely to get sick in the first place and more likely to respond well to treatment. It has also been found that if you change the meaning of stress itself from a negative to a positive (stress is your body's way of preparing you for action) then the effects are mitigated.[42]

Measurement of Stress; Heart Rate variability

The heart has always been understood to be an organ that is affected by stress – the heart rate invariably increases under stress in preparation for action, for instance. What is less well known is that the difference between heart beats, **Heart Rate Variability (HRV)**, can be a very accurate indicator of the unconscious stress that the body is under. This is controlled by its innervation (nerve input) by the three branches of the autonomic

---

people cycle in and out in the early stages of their illness and then end up stuck in a preferential state of fight and flight or freeze.

nervous system, via the vagus nerve. When the body is in homeostasis (more correctly called '**allostasis**' in current biological understanding) these opposing control systems are in perfect balance so that if you need to gear up for action the sympathetic system is stimulated and when you need to calm down the parasympathetic systems come to the fore. Interestingly the heart beat registers the balance between these every time you breathe in and out. The in breath is stimulatory (sympathetic) and the out breath is calming/relaxing (parasympathetic). This is why we use breathwork a lot in modulating stress arousal (see later chapter).

The heart registers this finely tuned balance by its variability, the beat to beat gap which should vary in a regular way depending how well your ANS is working. The body is designed to be able to dynamically adjust itself to perform optimally within a defined range of stimuli. Amongst others, the Institute of Heart Math, a US-based organisation, has been researching this interesting marker and quotes: "a number of studies have shown that HRV is an important indicator of both physiological resiliency and behavioural flexibility, reflecting an individual's capacity to adapt effectively to stress and environmental demands"[43]. It is the basis for much biofeedback treatment (see later chapter). Note it is not the same as your heartbeat, it is a measurement of the variation in the beat to beat distance. The output can be shown to vary hugely depending on your mental state:

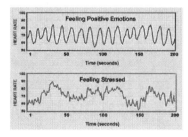

Figure 13 Heart Rate Variability

This used to be something you could only measure when hooked up to a specialised electrocardiogram (ECG) machine but happily this is now made a lot easier by simple free 'apps' that you can download onto your smartphone or tablet. I have used the most readily available free one, HeartMonitor and, although I cannot vouch for its accuracy compared to a professional machine, as a relative tool for marking your stress levels it is brilliant as you can take different measurements at different times in your life. For instance, I measured mine after a stressful day at work (where my day is not my own but I am subject to the deadlines and priorities of others) compared to a day at my clinic with my clients. The differences were startling – a 50% difference. HRV is a powerful, objective and non-invasive tool to measure your body's finely tuned hormonal, behavioural responses to the day to day stresses. I urge you to measure yours, in states of stress and relaxation initially, to see for yourself how this varies. The next stage is to actually be able to dynamically altering the output by 'focusing' on trying to make the waves increase in amplitude (height) and become more regular. It is worth trying for yourself to see if you can control your HRV by learning to tune into it. This is biofeedback in action which we cover in more detail in Section Four.

We have long known that the heart is an intuitive organ – we understand that things are 'heartfelt', and a broken heart is what we feel if we are very sad. These colloquial terms are not just random, they express what we have always known, that the heart with its central importance to health and wellbeing, often senses things *before the brain*[44]. Indeed, "the heart has its own intrinsic nervous system that operates and processes information independently of the brain or nervous system"[45]. This is what enables a heart transplant to work before the vagus nerve is fully functional. It is also an endocrine organ producing oxytocin, the bonding hormone with others. Its electromagnetic field is large and is largely responsible for allowing us to attune to other people (or not!). It is an organ of coherence; when its electromagnetic rhythm is in harmony with others we feel at ease and at peace with the world. This is the desired outcome of all meditative endeavours and is an essential pre-requisite to fully achieve health and wellbeing. The origin of coherence is in the heart and its connection with the brain is specifically the amygdala which it innervates via its **afferent** (towards the brain) nerves. You can see therefore another instance of the mind-body connection in operation that we are only now beginning to ascertain. In these activities and its vital pumping action it is no surprise that the heart uses a lot of energy. It has the highest energy requirement second to the brain and is very densely packed with mitochondria which we will turn to now.

Mitochondria and Energy production; a survival response

Energy production in the cell

So let's return to what happens in the cell in chronic illness set in motion by a highly stressed system. Once a cycle of oxygen deprivation from stress activation is established, other effects naturally follow. When a tissue is deprived of oxygen it will start to become difficult to meet your energy requirements because oxygen is needed for energy production. The molecule of energy storage and release is called **ATP** (**adenosine tri-phosphate** - think of it as energy 'currency') – it is constantly being broken down to **ADP** (**adenosine diphosphate**) with the release of a phosphate molecule and energy and then recycled back to ATP[54]. See below:

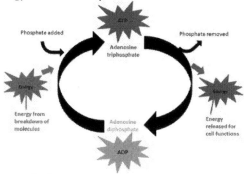

Figure 14 The Energy Cycle

However, if the tissue is not able to respire properly (due to stress, low oxygen or toxicity) ATP recycling becomes slowed and we enter a phase of anaerobic respiration (without oxygen). In order to meet the oxygen requirements of the tissue then the body has to turn to a secondary anaerobic pathway (called **glycolysis**) which releases lactic acid as a by-product – the same molecule that causes cramp in athletes if they run out of oxygen through overworking a particular muscle. This secondary pathway is highly inefficient compared to the oxygen requiring pathway (respiration) – it only produces 2 ATP compared to 34 in the oxygen requiring pathway. It is meant to be a temporary addition or stopgap only.

With chronic conditions of cell stress however, this deprivation does not go away; stress alters the balance in the cell towards the more inefficient pathway. In fact as people try to 'push through' the problem they only compound the issue of oxygen deficit. Eventually, you may enter a phase in which even the anaerobic cycle cannot supply enough ATP and you run out of energy completely – we see this for example in chronic fatigue style syndromes which we discuss in more detail later.

Allied with this is a failure of the hormone balance system; specifically the thyroid and adrenals. These two systems lie at the heart of most chronic disease. Both require metabolic energy, which as we've seen is one of the

---

54 Traditionally we have thought the energy comes from the release of the chemical energy of the phosphate bond when it is broken. This turns out to be incorrect as we shall see later.

components that is most at risk when the body is in fight, flight or freeze. This has systemic consequences; the brain will slow thought processes such as memory and ability to focus become impaired (referred to as 'brain fog'). The body will show symptoms of dry skin, thinning hair, pallor (or flushing depending on which system is the most depleted – low thyroid tends towards paleness), tiredness unrelieved by rest, allergies, etc. Without wishing to sound grandiose, I can tell low thyroid signs just by looking. People with this condition tend to have a puffy, pale, dry look to their skin, thinning hair, with often poor tolerance of exercise. It is extremely common in women over 50 and very highly implicated in the development of chronic illness. The body needs energy for every function, including, of course, to keep itself warm; a low body temperature, therefore, acts as a reliable sign of low metabolic energy. I use it clinically.

The thyroid gland, at the base of the neck, makes the hormone **T4 (thyroxine)** with four iodine molecules. T4 converts to **T3 (triiodothyronine)** and **RT3 (reverse T3)** with 3 molecules controlled by a chemical reaction that requires Selenium and an abundance of B-vitamins. If you are depleted in these as most of us are then the reactions cannot take place efficiently and hypothyroidsim will result. Less T3 or more RT3 (a metabolic dead end of poor conversion) slows down energy production, and fatigue and poor immune system function are the result. In short you feel lousy. Production of these thyroid hormones is controlled by **TSH (Thyroid Stimulating Hormone)**, from the pituitary gland and then via the hypothalamus which as we've seen is highly implicated in the stress response. So you can see how stress might impact on hormonal balance and energy production in the body. Now we need to look in more detail at where this energy deprivation all happens.

Mitochondrial dysfunction

Mitochondria are the basic power-houses of the cell that belie our evolutionary origins. About 2 billion years ago a unicellular organism (called an Archaea) engulfed a bacterium to create the first ever multi-cellular (eukaryotic) organism. This is the ancestor of our cells today with mitochondria being the remnants of that bacterium. You may even think they look quite like one – it's true they do and this is why. Notice the convoluted membranes which increase the surface area for chemical reactions (much like your intestines wrap around inside you).

Figure 15. A Cell Mitochondrion

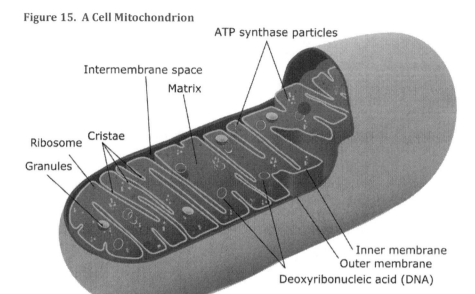

For many years mitochondrial energy production has been described as being the result of transfers of electrons along a chain of molecules called the **electron transport chain (ETC)** on the inner membrane of the mitochondrion. This structure straddles the mitochondrial inner membrane which, like all biological membranes, is composed of a 2-layer lipid (fat) sandwich which keeps the fluids on 2 sides separate. The mitochondrial membrane is particularly adapted to energy production and has a series of molecular protein complexes which use a flow of electrons (small charged particles on the outside of each atom) to engineer a sequence of chemical reactions leading to the production of ATP (remember the' energy 'currency' of the cell). This sequence was traditionally conveyed rather like an engine, with a piston at the end (the ATP synthase molecule). However we now know that this machine-based idea is wildly inaccurate and fails to highlight the incredible complexity of mitochondrial function. The mitochondrion is a "dynamic organ responding to the needs of its environment by organising electron flow to optimise the use of available substrates"[46]. It is able to sense the environment in minute detail and adapt its function accordingly. It is very far from a machine, at least not any machine that man has ever made.

It has long been known that plants are able to harness light energy via the green chlorophyll molecule that they contain. But it is only in the last couple of years or so that mammalian cells have been shown to also harvest light via molecules such as adenine (in ATP), many of the molecules in the unsaturated fats such as **docosahexanoic acid** (**DHA**), and chlorophyll and other molecules from the diet. So, the textbook definition of mitochondrial function needs to be re-written; far from being merely a conveyer belt of electrons it is the energy of *photons* that are actually being harnessed via the electromagnetic resonance of certain molecules in the chain. The double bonds of molecules such as the adenine in ATP allow an electromagnetic field to create an electron flow of incredible speed (about 10^{14}). Here is a diagram of the flow of information (light, electrons (and protons shown as H+). Light is not shown in the diagram as I couldn't yet find any images that included it but it interacts at the **cytochromeC** (**CytC**) stage (between complex III and IV).

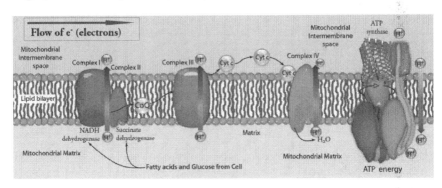

Figure 16. The Electron Transport Chain (ETC) of the Mitochondrial membrane

Photons, it seems, are the source of information flow in the body not electrons. This is a radical new understanding. Mitochondria are the organelles of cell-light interaction and light itself may be the information code (harnessed also by DNA which contains the same adenine molecule as one of its bases). Certain molecules like ATP and haem (in hameoglobin the oxygen-holding moleclule of red blood cells) or chlorophyll act as antennae to light or **chromophores**. Certain plant nutrients like polyphenols (e.g. resveratrol in red wine, CoenzymeQ10 (coQ10), DHA (a fatty acid found in fish oil), and curcumin from turmeric are also light harvesting due to their alternating double bonds[55]. Here are some biological chromophores:

---

[55] This may explain why these molecules are particularly health promoting as they enable more energy production and better signalling (communication) between molecules.

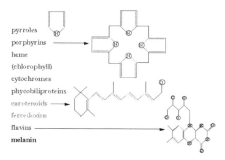

pyrroles
porphyrins
heme
(chlorophyll)
cytochromes
phycobiliproteins
carotenoids
ferredoxins
flavins
melanin

Figure 17 Biolgocial Chromophores

Note the preponderance of double bonds between atoms (which create electron clouds around them); a ring structure is powerful. Something of particular interest to biologists is the similarity between chlorophyll (the molecule responsible for photosynthesis in plants) and haem (the molecule that carries oxygen in the blood of animals): the only difference is Magnesium (Mg) is at the centre in plants and Iron (Fe) in haem. Interesting isn't it?

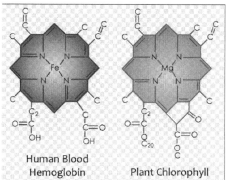

Human Blood Hemoglobin   Plant Chlorophyll

Figure 18. Haemoglobin and Chorophyll

We have long known this structural similarity. But until now we did not realise that similar mechanisms of light harvesting occur in both animals and plants. We assumed that plants did the light harvesting and we converted plant energy by eating them. The reality is that we use plant molecules more directly via photon harvesting. We co-evolved with plants so it is no surprise to me that plant based molecules can enhance human metabolic function. However, the recent discovery that "dietary metabolites of chlorophyll can enter the circulation, are present in tissues, and can be enriched in the mitochondria where they increase the ATP production of cells"[47] is completely new. It is highly accelerated electrons (from the energy harvested from a passing photon) that make such high production of energy possible not the release of chemical energy from the breaking of chemical bonds as we formerly believed. This vastly more efficient and dynamic energy release "stimulated the evolution of the nervous system and brain" via the chromophore properties of the fatty acid **Decosahexanoic Acid (DHA)** which enabled us to "evolve from unicellular organisms into the complex multi-cellular organisms we are[48]. These quantum phenomena of information flow are only now beginning to be understood and incorporated into textbooks[49.] You will struggle to find mention of light harvesting in humans; indeed, I thought they were only 'new age' understandings until I heard this from well respected nutritional scientist and checked the literature. This is not science fiction, it is science fact.

What is important for us is that mitochondria are intelligent, dynamic organelles which can respond to the environment. When the cell senses a threat called it activates the **Cell Danger Response (CDR)**, the aerobic (oxygen-using) respiration is down-regulated and our cells shift to an alternative pathway outside the mitochondria which is anaerobic and produces much less ATP from glucose (the sugar that we burn). This means less energy is available for all the work of the cell; repair, renewal, cell signalling and protein manufacture. The cell goes on a 'go slow' and if the CDR does not abate the cell becomes fixed in this pattern which is highly dangerous for the organism (us). We will see later how this relates to certain chronic illnesses, but for now the main thing to understand is that failure of the mitochondria (**mitochondriopathy**) is at the heart of most chronic disease[50] and *reversing the message of threat is the priority in recovery.*

Chapter 5: Mind and Memory

Conscious versus Subconscious process (mind)

So far we have looked at the structures of the brain involved in the survival response (limbic system) and areas that control them. It is less clear at the moment where in the brain the areas of conscious and unconscious processing are. The 'unconscious mind', as described by psychologists from Freud onwards, was thought to be the holy grail of understanding of the mind until the recent advent of cognitive behavioural models. However as a metaphor for working with the mind, it still has application, particularly in the area of hypnotherapy and some forms of psychotherapy which utilise it.

The unconscious part of the mind is by far the larger and is, in fact, the dominant part, constantly assessing our environment and adjusting the internal processes and indeed our behaviours, without our conscious involvement. It corresponds to the primary survival areas of the brain which develop in the human at an earlier age than the cortex. You may have seen the familiar 'iceberg' model of the mind where most is under the surface, of course this is only a metaphor but at least it portrays to people the relative sizes of the two processes.

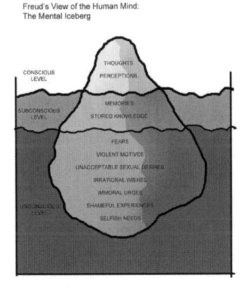

Freud's View of the Human Mind:
The Mental Iceberg

CONSCIOUS LEVEL

THOUGHTS
PERCEPTIONS

SUBCONSCIOUS LEVEL

MEMORIES
STORED KNOWLEDGE

UNCONSCIOUS LEVEL

FEARS
VIOLENT MOTIVES
UNACCEPTABLE SEXUAL DESIRES
IRRATIONAL WISHES
IMMORAL URGES
SHAMEFUL EXPERIENCES
SELFISH NEEDS

Figure 19. The Mental Iceberg

Although we consider it a metaphor; as there is no one area of the brain that correlates absolutely to the 'unconscious' it is generally understood to be the more evolutionarily primitive parts. Freud considered there to be three levels and he made a distinction between the unconscious and the subconscious. Perhaps best thought of as mapping to the brainstem and limbic system respectively, there are many subtleties of connection that this model ignores. It may be more correct to think about the unconscious *process* of mind not parts of the brain. If you are at all confused about the distinction between brain and mind (as I have been as they are frequently confused in common usage) then think of mind as what the brain *does*. Mind is the combination of all the processes occurring in the brain from the automatic regulation of the body, through memory storage to consciousness itself (and don't get me started on the controversy around what consciousness is!). Some have described the mind as more of a mindbody phenomenon that 'interpenetrates the brain and body with photons of light held in an energy field'. The molecule DHA (remember this is a chromophore) may be the molecule that underpins this quantum electromagnetic effect[48]. Although this is not common understanding it is beginning to be recognised that light may be the basic 'currency' of the universe, and certainly the vibration of light constitutes electromagnetic energy which permeates all things[51]. We have seen already how important this is in energy creation within the cell. We can now turn to how the mind organises perception and beliefs within this energetic understanding.

The **conscious mind** is the volitional or thinking mind, it analyses and judges – it's the problem-solver. It is the site of the short-term or working memory – where you control your current activity – this has limits (which are generally believed to be 5 or 6 things to be kept in working memory at any one time for approximately 20 seconds). The *conscious* mind is the part that controls our reasoning ability, our short-term memory and our will-power. It is the part we use to solve problems and analyse our everyday experience and it is time-bound. We spend most of our time thinking about what happened in the past or agonising about the future! It is however, the smallest part of our mind; so possesses the least important functions for our bodily experience.

The **subconscious or unconscious mind** (perhaps corresponding to the limbic system and brainstem) is the seat of our long-term memories and belief system. Everything that has ever happened to you is stored there[27]. Interestingly though, it is timeless; everything is in the perpetual present there – a feature that is important with trauma as we will see. It also controls all of our automatic functions – our breathing, heart rate, etc which we don't have to consciously think about so could be said consist of the primitive reptilian brain or brain stem. It is responsible for controlling basic essential functions without our awareness. It may also be the site of our intuition or 'gut feelings'. This has probably given us an evolutionary advantage as, if all our brain power were taken up with thinking about breathing and the beating of our heart, there would have been very little left to know when to run from the sabre-toothed tiger now approaching us! Clearly there is an advantage to having the most basic functions running 'behind the scenes' without us having to think about it. The unconscious mind is habitual and automatic – it monitors the body and compares what's going on to what it has met before. It is literal but it communicates via emotions and symbols i.e. it is sensory based and its role is to keep you safe.

The important part is that most of us are running on unconscious programmes over which we have very little control. Hence you will have noticed that some things that you do you don't even remember doing or do automatically (e.g. driving a familiar route) or, more importantly for our discussion, habitual behaviours, have been downloaded from our experience, particularly in our childhood. In fact these habits of behaviour have become so ingrained in our personality structures (themselves a construct of experience) that we take them completely for granted; they are unconscious too. Remember, it is the not the events themselves that necessarily create the unconscious response but our interpretation of them which varies according to our beliefs (perceptions) of their importance/ threat.

Belief Systems

Bruce Lipton, in his ground-breaking book 'The Biology of Belief[52]' showed us how it is the filter of our perception that not only determines our behaviour but our *physiology too* via the selective expression of our genes (epigenetics). He and many others have shown us that genes are not destiny. Beliefs are far more important. If you believe that you are going to get cancer because you mother had it (the belief only has to be an unconscious fear not something you'd consciously vocalise) then your thoughts can actually influence physiology to make it so. We will return to this idea later in the field of chronic pain.

The unconscious is also the site of our values and belief systems. It is the fact that it is unconscious which makes it so difficult for us to perceive the origins of our own behaviour – we simply are unaware of why we act the way we do. However, I would suggest that we *always* know when we are working contrary to our values and beliefs. Our emotions, often expressed in our bodies, tell us when we are in internal conflict. The problem is we are often not attuned to hearing these messages, we bury them in work or other diversions to avoid feeling them; that is how illness or 'dis-ease' may result.

Speaking to this part of our mind must be done in the present tense as it works in a timeless zone where past and future don't exist. This is the problem with many people's use of affirmations to effect change. They will say 'I can be happy', 'I will lose weight', and although positive thinking has its benefits (it helps to rebalance the overall negative bias of the thinking brain for instance), it seldom achieves as much as we hoped. The subconscious hears 'I will' as the future tense and says 'ok, nothing to do here then as it's not happening now'. When working hypno-therapeutically with clients it is important to get them to act like the thing they want is already here. So, the statement becomes 'I am healing', even though they may not feel it yet, just the act of saying something makes it possible for the subconscious to set that in motion. We use the power of imagination to create the possibility 'in the now'. You will see more of that in action in the case study section.

Since your values and beliefs are what drive your behaviour it is no use frankly deciding to do something that you subconscious does not agree with. It will subtly subvert you. Ever determined that you were going to lose weight, become fitter, get a better job, etc but found you lost motivation before you achieved your goal? Well what may be going on is that under the surface, unbeknown to you is that it is going against something that you unconsciously believe. For me, for instance, leaving a secure job to become self-employed is going against my belief that security is important and risk is dangerous (I have, I think, put that one to rest!). Some people's belief systems are inherited from their parents, or peers without ever having been consciously examined. When we do therapy together, clients often report they 'had absolutely no idea' they believed certain things, until they come up during interactions with their subconscious mind.

Finally, even the iceberg metaphor may be huge understatement in terms of processing power. If we think of the mind as a computer then, the conscious mind can process 2,000 bits of information per second (which allows us to keep 3- 4 things happening at the same time – women more than men). But the subconscious in contrast has an astounding 4 billion bits per second of processing power so you can see the ration is 2 million :1. An astounding difference! No wonder then that we need to harness the power of the unconscious to effect change. But there is another level of complexity pertinent to our discussion– the brain is divided into two halves that operate differently.

Left and Right hemispheres

The different functions of the left and right hemispheres of the brain, specifically the cortex or thinking brain have been popularised by the media as being 'you're a left brain or right brain person' but that is not strictly accurate. All people use both sides (although perhaps to different degrees). The model shown below is based on a right handed person so for left-handed people you would need to swap this model round.

Table 4 The Left and Right Hemispheres

Left Hemisphere	Right hemisphere
Logic	Imagination
Words	Pictures
Parts	Whole
Analysis (breaks apart)	Synthesise (puts things together)
Order/ control	Spontaneity/freedom

Obviously we need both to function well and the quality of the inter-hemispherical dialogue is vital. Thankfully in a human there is part of the brain that controls this dialogue. The **corpus callosum (CC)** is a bundle of nerve fibres that acts as a communication pathway between the two hemispheres – this tends to happen when you are in 'the flow' of awareness and good feelings; the crosstalk is good and you function well. You want to perceive reality through both hemispheres at the same time to analyse the most information and be able to react accordingly. When under stress this system may break down and you will naturally tend towards one side or the other, whichever has become typically dominant in you. This tendency towards one side or another becomes habitual and will be developed early without your conscious control.

So it's the wiring between the two sides via the CC that 'adds dimension and depth to everything you think and do'[53]. Contrary to popular opinion we are not either /or left-brain or right-brain people although our habitual tendency will be to defer one way or another. Interestingly men and women's brains are quite different in this respect. Women's' brains are more symmetrical with a stronger, thicker CC meaning that words (left-brain) carry more emotional meaning (right brain) for women than they do men. That would explain a lot I can hear you saying! Male brain's are more inclined to be left hemisphere dominant so they are good at logic and analysis (although of course there are variations in this).

Within each of the hemispheres there are some networks of neurons with specific functions and attributes. These are sometimes called 'modules' or networks by neurologists. Modules wire together and become more dominant as a result. We will see how this happens later. The important thing to remember here is that *mind is a process*, a result of the physiology (and quantum function) of the brain. It is *plastic* (alterable) because it is a result of neuronal connections that are dynamic in nature. You can change how you think. But let's look in more detail at the structure so we can understand the complexity of the brain.

The Role of the Prefrontal Cortex (PFC)

The region of the brain called the **prefrontal cortex (PFC)** is really what defines us as human; it is crucial for how we pay attention, it enables us to put things in the "front of our mind" and hold them in awareness. It is the basis of our moral system and capacity for empathy. It is likely that this in an area that certain groups of people e.g. therapists (!) have highly developed (initially by environmental exposure and then by training). Studies of people who have suffered injury to the PFC show us that it is an important brain area for creating our 'map of the world' i.e. the mental representation of our outer experience. Various different parts of the cortex have specific functions:

Figure 20 The Pre-Frontal Cortex (PFC) regions in the two hemispheres

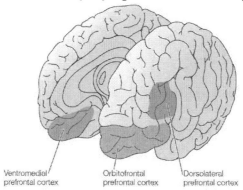

Ventromedial prefrontal cortex   Orbitofrontal prefrontal cortex   Dorsolateral prefrontal cortex

The **Medial Pre-frontal Cortex (MPFC)** is the integration centre involved in co-ordinating left and right sides with direct connections to the amygdala in the limbic system). This part is importantly involved in our sense of curiosity and awareness and is the part that we target in therapy particularly for dissociated clients who have lost connection with their bodily self. It is activated during mindfulness meditation or mindful awareness or psychotherapy.

The **Dorso-lateral Pre-frontal cortex (DPFC)** is the site of our short-term or working memory and has no direct connection with the limbic system. It is the last bit to develop in the human and often the first to go with ageing. We've all had the experience of walking into a room and forgetting why we went there – this is a failure of this part of the brain to hold the requisite information for long enough for us to commit it to longer term memory

The **Right Orbital Pre-frontal cortex (ROPFC)** (so called because it is directly behind the right orbit of the eye) is most specifically concerned with emotions and arousal regulation as it has good connections with the limbic system and can inhibit activation. It develops early in life and is the social centre of the brain, which, if given support and trusting relationships in those early years, becomes more capable of regulating emotion but it depends on good parental attachment as investigators Allan Shore and others have shown)[54]. It could be seen as our 'soothing centre' if it is promoted by secure attachment. We have all seen examples of people for whom this is not the case and how 'up and down' or entirely absent their emotions can be. Our prisons are full of such people where auto-regulation has never been learnt.

Through its links with the limbic system, and the immune system via regulating levels of cortisol, it acts as the interface between mind and body and so is implicated in unexplained medical complaints such as fibromyalgia or pelvic pain which are the body's way of expressing emotions through pain. This is called **somatisation**. Defined as feeling emotions through the body rather than as feelings, these issues are common in people "in whom emotion is undifferentiated and unregulated"[55]. In other words they can't tell one emotion from another and they may find it difficult to put words to feelings; memories may also be completely dissociated from feelings. I met one such person who was on a training course with me. He described some awful events that happened in his childhood without emotion of any kind. He, I now know, is suffering from **alexithymia** which could be seen as a failure of the ROPFC. Somatisation is not a commonly understood concept although, in fact, it lies at the base of many of the chronic pain syndromes I am exploring in this book. It is a direct example of how poor relationships and unexpressed emotions make us ill.

The cortex is known to go 'offline' in the aftermath of trauma which may explain the hyper/hypo arousal of PTSD as the cortex is normally the modulator of experience, helping to bring logic and a 'wider view' . In trauma work we often talk about 'getting curious' as the antidote to these limbic states. We need to engage people in what happens when they think a certain thought or act a certain way, get them tuning in to their body states – something that they may have actively blocked from childhood onwards.

When you begin to look at your reactions as symptoms (i.e "I've been triggered and this is my survival brain in charge") and not from an underlying pathology (i.e. I'm mad, bad or weak), you begin to see how extraordinary the human brain is and your curiosity (MFPC-mediated) is aroused[56]. This is a direct antidote to the dissociation and emotional dampening that many people suffer after a traumatic experience. It is the direct target of intervention, whether by linking the two sides of the cortex as in EMDR or by hypnotherapy and CBT whereby we engage the imagination and the thinking brain respectively. We cover these therapies on more detail in the last section. Suffice to say there is an answer, these states can be reversed; the brain is plastic.

Interactions between the cortex and the limbic system; the anterior cingulate and insula

There is another important part of the mid-brain (adjacent to the amygdala) that has a function in registering threat and helping to lay the foundations of trauma. It's called the **Anterior cingulate cortex (ACC)** and is important as a filtering system. It is another part of the brain that is wiped out as a result of trauma[57]. It possesses structures called spindle cells which wrap around the nerve bundle of fibres linking the left to the right sides of the brain. This may be very important for how emotions are integrated and meaning made of the emotional events in our lives.

The ACC is primarily involved in fear conditioning as it normally inhibits the amygdala, which as we know is the primary area for threat encoding. However, it also appears to play a role in emotionality, selective attention, and certain social functions, including emotional attachments and parenting, as well as generation of the concept of the self in relation to society. It is my contention that this is the part of the brain that fails in attachment disorder, and other more chronic trauma disorders. I have particularly noticed that the sense of self is often highly distorted, even in very outwardly functional people. They operate despite their own self-loathing to become very respected/hard-working/ achieving people but when questioned they cannot see that anything they have done has any worth. If you press them they will acknowledge grudgingly that it might have value but they do not feel that emotionally, it is more of an intellectual

---

56 The opposite of what most people experience when they enter the medical system for help with a mental health issue. The process of labelling the disease and pathologising the person creates more stress as they wonder what they did to deserve such a thing and is deeply shamed by being ill.

57 For many years it was considered part of the mammalian limbic system along with the amygdala. However, more recently this has been called into question and it is thought to be more of an adaptation of the cortex46

awareness. The ACC might be the bit that we bring 'online' when we target memories in trauma treatment as when we do EMDR. We rewire the responses by a process of *extinguishing* the conditioned response. More on that later.

The **insula** (another part of the cortex just behind the PFC) is an area that helps interpret incoming sensation, rating it dangerous or not. It is highly involved in our subjective experience of pain, for example, and can become active just by imagining pain as well as in more pleasant experiences like music appreciation. It monitors incoming signals from the body (particularly the physiological experience of emotions like sadness, fear, anger, etc) and combines this information with the limbic system and brainstem to generate appropriate responses. As we will see later, when the signals get scrambled by unresolved emotional memory, stress hits the 'play' button and all incoming signals are interpreted as painful, dangerous or life-threatening, causing all sorts of chronic pain and stress-related diseases.

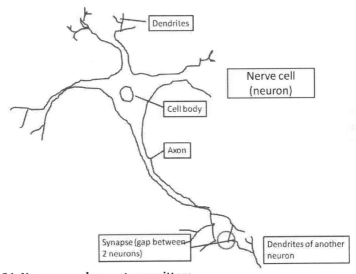

Figure 21. Neurons and neurotransmitters

Neurons are nerve cells that conduct information signals throughout the body. The important part of the nerve in terms of control of what information is passed on and how quickly is the synapse which is shown above. This is the gap between the axons of one cell and the dendrites of another. The signal is both electrical (there has to be a voltage difference

111

between one side and the other – called an 'action potential' – which creates the electrical charge difference with allows the neurotransmitters and peptides to pass across the gap where they are picked up by the appropriate receptors. The chemical message is like a key fitting within a lock and once it is picked up by the receptor it triggers a downstream response of more activity. When many neurons are connected in this way a signal is conducted through them like a signal along a wire.

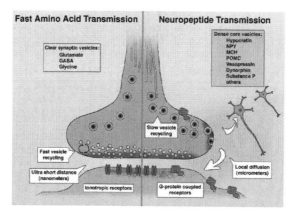

Figure 22 Neurotransmitters compared

However, that's a highly simplified version of what really happens which I am not going to go into here. Suffice to say the synapse is where the 'action is' and its efficiency is controlled by a number of chemicals secreted into the gap – both **neurotransmitters** and **neuropeptides** (small proteins).

Out of around 80 neurotransmitters that we know of the vast majority of nerve impulses are facilitated by just two; **glutamate** – an excitatory molecule and **Gamma-Aminobutyric acid (GABA)** – an inhibitory one. As with many systems in the body there are many checks and balances within the system. The other main transmitters[58], more properly called **neuromodulators** because their function is more to modulate the effect of the others via altering the sensitivity of the synaptic receptors. Of the three main ones that are important to our discussion there are:

- **Dopamine (DA)** which sharpens and focuses attention i.e. it enhances *vigilance*

---

58 . The neuropeptides were only discovered in the last 30 years of so whereas neurotransmitters have been known about a lot longer. See 'Molecules of Emotion' by Candace Pertl.

- **Serotonin (S)** which alters the *emotional tone* of a signal
- **Noradrenaline (NA** or Norepinephrine) which amplifies a signal i.e. *significance*

Substance P

One neuropeptide that deserves special mention here is **Substance P (SP)** is a neuropeptide produced in the spinal cord and also in the limbic system. It used to be regarded as the main neurotransmitter involved in the transmission of pain (hence the 'P') as it as shown to increase sensitivity to pain. Recently, however, research has found that it is a neuromodulator involved in other aspects of sensory response such as emotional regulation, and involved in the integration of pain, stress, and anxiety. It has been found that "emotional stressors increase SP efflux in specific limbic structures such as amygdala and septum and that the magnitude of this effect depends on the severity of the stressor"[56]. So this could explain why pain itself is a stressor and adds to the anxiety response. It has been shown to trigger inflammatory histamine release from mast cells and cause oedema, vomiting and restless leg syndrome which may account for these symptoms in long term pain syndromes. For a long time it was considered central in the development of fibromyalgia, a condition of persistent pain which we look at later where increased levels of SP in the spinal cord might cause a heightened awareness of pain. This might explain the main feature of fibromyalgia which is **allodynia** where a non-painful touch stimulus is perceived by the body as being intensely painful.

Neuroplasticity and sensitisation

It used to be thought that the neurons you were born with were the same number you died with. In other words that once your brain was fully formed it would never change its neural pathways. Now we know that simply isn't true. With the spectacular advance in brain imaging technology (particularly via **functional MRI (fMRI)** we can see that neuronal pathways are constantly changing – new neurons being formed in areas of high usage and new neural connections lighting up when we start to think or behave in novel ways. So, the brain is not a static transmitter but an organic filtering station, constantly responding to input and altering its function to suit. There is a lovely phrase 'what fires together wires together' which means that when certain pathways light up the chain of neurons becomes more established and easier to fire next time. In other words the brain is adapting to its environment and what is needed to make the process more energy efficient and more automatic. This is termed **neuroplasticity**.

This has positive and negative effects. On the positive side it enables us to do relatively straightforward functions like driving and operating machinery without having to think too hard about it. We can even develop our skills to become highly proficient at creative acts like dancing and playing the piano. This is why we need to practice as – the converse of the adage above 'use it or lose it' is in indeed true. Neuroplasticity is also "what makes memory possible'[53]. We would be unable to record anything new if we couldn't wire new connections.

However, on the negative side, if we are depressed, constantly thinking about bad things that may happen or we find that certain things trigger us to anxiety, these neural networks become reinforced. Repetition rewires the brain via something called **long term potentiation** (**LTP**); the more they fire, the more efficient they get and this breeds habits of thinking and behaviour. So the more you think something (a habitual thought) the easier it becomes to think those things over and over again. We become stuck in a negative cycle. Fear based thoughts are particularly difficult to eradicate as we've seen, as they are encoded in the emotional brain so that they never decay (a survival mechanism to avoid something in future). Howard Schubiner calls it our "emotional speed dial because our bodies can typically react to emotional triggers before we are even aware of the trigger"[70].

So thoughts and hence behaviour changes the structure of the brain in an organic fashion; responding to the needs of the (perceived) environment. Interestingly, however so does imagining those same behaviours via 'behavioural rehearsal'. This is familiar to us as we know an anxious mind will replay over and over again possible scenarios. We can use it positively however, in therapy where we encourage you to invent a new, more positive outcome and we get you to replay that over and over again until the neural pathways are reinforced whilst the old connections are de-potentiated. This is particularly powerful in the relaxed state of hypnosis (more about that in Section Four).

Interestingly, when you develop new ideas or insight, change in the brain occurs more quickly than when you learn a new language because of special structures in the brain called **spindle cells**. These are specialised thickened nerve fibres which create a unique interface between thoughts and emotions by integrating information from neural pathways (called 'neural nets' that you have already formed. They therefore allow you to make quick leaps in understanding. I have witnessed this when performing therapy with people – their face changes as they make the connection. I call it the 'ah-ha' moment. This is a way we can encourage people to move forward in therapy e.g. to 'unlearn' their pain which has become an over-sensitised default pathway.

Memory and consolidation

Memory is not a 'thing' even though we talk about it as such. It is a *process* driven by neural networks (neurones which link together in distinct relationships). We have seen that the more certain pathways fire, the easier it gets to stimulate them. And that the opposite is also true; lesser used pathways become defunct. However now we wish to turn to how memories are formed and stored. During trauma certain pathways are highly stimulated, the body is flooded with stress hormones; adrenaline, noradrenaline and cortisol from your adrenals, and glutamate which prime the amygdala to 'code' the event as dangerous. This inhibits the functioning of the hippocampus which normally date stamps the memory and stores it in the appropriate neural networks - **memory consolidation**. Under trauma therefore the normal memory consolidation process is hijacked[57]. Memories remain as fragments unavailable to conscious or narrative recall for many years – they have become *implicit* within the amygdala and other deep brain regions. They also become your default pathways, even when the stimulus is not so life threatening. In other words they become habitual.

These implicit memories are coded by the emotional brain with associations; sensations (sight, sound, feeling), the emotions felt at the time the event happens and a belief system that goes with it (which may be a wordless sense of shame or fear initially but over time and repetition becomes so embedded it becomes normal and part of our personality). Habitual reactions to these deep implicit memories become routine and unquestioned; we may even be unaware that we are reacting from these deeply held beliefs about ourselves. The more we do it, the more embedded the responses become, the less it becomes questioned. It thus has deep impact on the way we behave throughout our life unless it becomes disabling in which case we might wonder why and seek treatment.

Implicit memories have 3 characteristics that set them apart from 'normal' (i.e. explicit memories. They are:

1. Persistent: they do not decay with time but remain highly charged ready to be activated in case of threat to the self
2. Present – there is no concept of time in this primitive part of the brain. Everything feels as if it's happening NOW
3. Pervasive – because these emotional memories (and their symptoms – the so-called 'pathological fragments'[58]) have been coded as essential to survival they permeate our lives.

Interestingly even though there is no absolute sense of time within these implicit memories, something may code them to allow anniversaries to be triggered subconsciously. I had one client who found herself suffering terrible symptoms of PTSD one day for no reason only to realise later that it was exactly one year since terrible events had occurred. The subconscious systems had noticed that the date was the same even though she had not consciously made the connection.

Memory types.

Although memory is not a 'thing' that we can locate in specific parts of the brain it can be thought of as a series of neural connections which light up both when the event happens (storage) and when we recall it. We can conceive of it as a process of "changes in synaptic strength between (..) systems distributed throughout the brain"[59]. there are dominant pathways that we may identify as being involved. There are many different types of memory. The main distinction is between long-term and short-term.

   1. Short-term Memory

Short-term (working) memory is where we store what is happening now – it is process based and limited to a certain number of items and is therefore easily overwhelmed. Unless we somehow add meaning to the information, or repeat it over again, it is usually lost within about 20 seconds. Doesn't say much our ability to keep things in mind does it! It is stored in the networks of the prefrontal cortex (PFC), the bit that humans have more of than other primates and which accounts for our (presumed) superior cognitive ability.

   2. Long-term memory

Within long-term memory there are a further two subtypes; **explicit** (sometimes called **declarative** i.e. verbal, language-based) and **implicit** (**non-declarative**) memory. What most people think of as a memory is the explicit memory is stored in the neural networks of the hippocampus (remember this is the date stamp or filing cabinet of the brain). It is subject to bias, in that we sometimes embellish or remove parts that don't 'fit' our beliefs, or map of the world. This is done subconsciously and we may not be aware we have mis-remembered and it becomes the truth as we know it.

Implicit vs. Explicit memory

Implicit memory (also called procedural memory) is the 'how' of doing something, an unconscious process stored within the cerebellum, caudate nucleus and parts of the motor cortex but mediated by the amygdala. For instance when you learnt to ride a bike this was the sort of memory that remembers how to do it for ever after. I have often found that these types of memories can be stored in the body as a wordless 'felt-sense' i.e. as a neuromuscular response controlled by the autonomic nervous system (mostly the branches of the vagus and other cranial nerves). It is this which is often triggered many years after trauma via body movements, flashbacks and other autonomic phenomena (panic attacks may be a specific flooding of the brain with implicit traumatic memory fragments). That these implicit memories are wordless, with no beginning, middle and end accounts for the fact that we often can't find language to describe what we are feeling. In cases such as these we need to approach the body rather than the mind when trying to access these memory fragments[23].

Implicit memory is the dominant type of memory prior to age 3 or 4 before our prefrontal cortex matures sufficiently and comes online. It explains why we have few specific memories that we can describe before this age. In many ways it is a survival response encoded to help us avoid a similarly dangerous experience in the future. It may have other names such as perceptual, muscle or body memory and has been approached using many successful body-oriented alternative therapies such as kinesiology. These approaches have been much derided as people make the mistake of thinking of all memory as being the more common explicit type and thus they miss the importance of this deeper type. As we shall see, sudden triggering of these implicit body memories may result in pain, tingling or dizziness which defy conventional thinking. It may even result in postural imbalances caused by chronic dissociation of parts of the body that were involved in a traumatic event. It is odd to think that pain or tension may be a memory but phantom limb pain (pain in a limb that has been lost) confirms that this is indeed possible.

Traumatic memory falls into this latter category as during trauma the hippocampus is turned down (by the release of cortisol) and the amygdala is enhanced thus implicit memory is more likely. Traumatic memory is, by its very nature, dissociated (recorded as sensory fragments without a narrative) as Bessel Van der Kolk has demonstrated[64]. Because it is largely dissociated we may not have a full recollection of the events that occurred and thus recall may be difficult or repressed entirely. It may seem strange to realise that such powerful events can be entirely forgotten but amnesia is in fact, a common correlate of trauma. There is plenty of evidence for this repression in accounts of childhood victims of abuse who have been recalled later in life to answer a standardised questionnaire on their sexual history. The study included questions about early sexual contact. A high number of the women questioned had no memory of the abuse for which they were hospitalised in their childhood – or the memories were subject to a reinterpretation – one woman described how she'd had an uncle who did something to another child but she told the story not as having happened to her but to someone else[60].

Many people, with less obvious traumas such as a difficult parental attachment, or bullying will deny they had any such history, not because they don't wish to admit it but because their mind has made it unavailable to conscious recall. Sometimes these memories may come up in fragments later in life as panic attacks or flashbacks (as in PTSD), or more commonly in lesser states by dizzy spells or by being flooded with pain [59]. They are the 'footprint' of implicit memory.

You may be triggered by all sorts of situations; people who unconsciously remind you of people or situations in your past, an association, look or smell. You may wonder why on earth you are reacting this way and this may lead you to question your history to the point where you will enter therapy to 'figure it all out'. If you are offered psychotherapy you may find you can analyse the reasons why you feel the way you do which will help somewhat but it may not change the way you feel because talking does not approach these implicit memories. For that we need access to the body (which reads the subconscious) as we will see.

This contradicts the notion that by describing our traumas we can somehow eradicate them and this is the major problem with conventional psychotherapies in the treatment of PTSD and other post-traumatic states. Talk therapies, of which CBT (cognitive behavioural therapy) is the current darling of the psychotherapy establishment, is very useful in many conditions – phobias, depression and anxiety being very well supported. But for conditions related to a traumatic memory (whether consciously or unconsciously held) it is of little value[38]. Indeed many have critiqued the CBT approach as being too limited in that not everything is a result of conscious thinking and so to base a therapy on 'reframing' thoughts does nothing to address the unconscious components of behaviour.

Moreover, to talk about the traumatic experience (as is the basis of most talk therapies) merely re-traumatises the holder of that memory as it experienced as happening 'now' not in the past. Because it has been has been coded as essential for survival it is still not able to be rationalised and 'pruned' as a normal memory would be i.e. the brain has no way of working out what part of the memory needs to be let go of. There are many crossovers here with addictions which are similarly coded and this is why they are so hard to give up with will-power alone. You are fighting a behaviour which your brain has stamped as essential to your survival using

---

59 Carolyn Spring, founder of the abuse survivor group, PODS describes suddenly having flashbacks and intrusions of memory in her thirties. Up to that point she felt she had had a normal childhood and life. She wondered if she was going mad but subsequent events proved her correct.

an extraordinarily hard-wired mechanism. The more you fight the feeling the harder it gets to overcome it as you enact your evolutionary biological imprint.

So when you get people to explore their implicit memories at first there may be very little that comes up except body sensations. Then without warning the feelings can then be so overwhelming that they trigger the person towards feelings of unsafety and disable the person completely. This can stop them from exploring these feelings (and the events they are tied to) both personally and in therapy. However, explore them you must if you are to overcome them. Luckily there are ways that the therapist can modulate the arousal; by stimulating bodily safety first then approaching, backing off, finding safety within, then approaching a little more, etc. This is called *pendulation* by Peter Levine, developer of Somatic sensing therapy and one of the first people to explore traumatic memory formation within the body.

The reason that traumatic memory is implicit (non-narrative) is that the stress arousal experienced at the time de-activates the frontal lobes which would normally inhibit the amgydala. The stress hormones then shrink the hippocampus which would help to code the memories as explicit/ verbal and give us the awareness that something is over and in the past. Trauma narrows down our experience and prevents us from processing our memories properly. In many ways your frontal lobes are your 'compassionate witness' which hears you and gives your story meaning. So a client without this ability feels constantly in danger as they can't process the memory out of unconscious storage – each time they are reminded of the event they are overwhelmed with feeling as if it is happening now. We will return to methods of releasing and processing these memories in therapy later. For now let's look at how the body deals with processing normal memories.

Rapid Eye Movement Sleep; memory consolidation
You may have wondered why you dream when you sleep. The latest research on dreams shows us that what we believed about sleep needs to be revised. We have known for about 50 years that dreams were important in 'pruning' memories i.e. analysing the events of our lives and discarding that information that is not needed and storing that which we may need to remember. It was noted that dreams coincided with a period of sleep called REM or Rapid eye movement sleep where the person would be visibly dreaming – the eyes would be moving under closed lids and sometimes the body would move a little too. Some people move more than others; sleep walking is phenomenon that demonstrates this[60].

Sleep is not a passive activity; recent research has found it to be a dynamic state of high activity and repair that runs through a cycle of 5 stages one of which is REM sleep. We seem to spend approximately 20% of our time in REM sleep (babies and infants spend nearly 50%[61]). We enter REM sleep more often in the later stages of sleep but it is in the transition between sleep states (REM and non-REM) that may hold the key to the healing properties of sleep[62] with the first being about neuronal recovery and the second being more to do with memory consolidation. The different stages seem to be signalled by the release of different neurotransmitters from the brain stem and different characteristic brain waves (electromagnetic) frequencies.

The initial stage of non-REM sleep, stage 1 is a very light stage from which we can be wakened easily. The eyes move slowly and muscle activity slows. If awakened from this stage we often report strange sensations and thoughts. We may 'jump' suddenly with a sensation of falling. Stage 2 begins when the brain wave activity slows and we enter a period of quieter muscle activity, this deepens in Stage 3 when delta waves[61] first appear, and take over almost exclusively in Stage 4. REM sleep is defined as the moment when we slip into irregular shallow breathing and rapid movements of the eyes. The amount of REM sleep we need will vary with our age and on how much we experienced the night before. If we are deprived of REM sleep it will be 'caught up' the following night with extended periods which shows how important it is. It seems to only occur in the higher mammals and not reptiles which suggests it may be involved in higher level cognitive functions such as memory consolidation, particularly the 'non-declarative, procedural and emotional memories[63]' that have such importance in trauma processing. It seems clear that REM sleep is necessary to our health but it may be the balance of the two (REM and Slow wave sleep or SWS) that is crucial. This is called the dual process hypothesis.

---

60 Some people have a condition known as xxx where the movements are not inhibited at all and they thrash about during sleep causing damage to themselves and things around them.

61 electrical activity of the brain at a frequency of around 1–8 Hz, typical of sleep. The resulting oscillations, detected using an electroencephalograph, are called delta waves.

Figure 22. Brain wave patterns

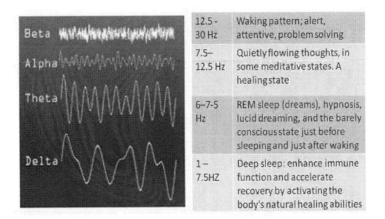

Beta	12.5 - 30 Hz	Waking pattern; alert, attentive, problem solving
Alpha	7.5– 12.5 Hz	Quietly flowing thoughts, in some meditative states. A healing state
Theta	6–7-5 Hz	REM sleep (dreams), hypnosis, lucid dreaming, and the barely conscious state just before sleeping and just after waking
Delta	1 – 7.5HZ	Deep sleep: enhance immune function and accelerate recovery by activating the body's natural healing abilities

Much is still to be learned but it is clear that certain disease states affect sleep as do some of the drugs used to treat them. Indeed for me, poor sleep was the first symptom to appear before all the others. I ignored it of course and carried on 'carrying on' as most of us do. Sleep hygiene (maintaining certain behaviours and light levels when sleeping, avoiding EMF exposure) is very important in regaining your health. But the main thing to help you sleep will be addressing the issues that are troubling you subconsciously. If you look at poor sleep as a message from your subconscious, something needs to be addressed. It may not be comfortable or convenient but you owe it to your health to stop avoiding and running from it.

CHAPTER 6: THE NATURE OF TRAUMA

Trauma is not always caused by the obvious large-scale events that most people perceive and understand it to be; in fact more or less anything can be traumatising if the person experiencing it has a degree of *powerlessness* at the time. And this is more likely when you are young. Bessel van der Kolk, the famous trauma researcher, devised a relationship between ability to recover and the age we are at when we first experience an event that we cannot escape and makes us feel helpless. He discovered indeed that there was an age / severity relationship but also that the more *betrayal* that is present at that event, the more difficult it is for us to recover. Betrayal is likely if the person who causes the trauma is someone you would expect to protect you. We see this especially in examples of abuse by parents for instance (which is much more common than anyone previously thought)[64].

However, bear in mind that *anything that induces shame* is experienced as trauma. This is an extremely important conclusion as all of us have some shame. The experience of shame is an important developmental stage which helps the infant brain to develop a sense of self. Shame signals from the mother in the first year of life identify behaviour which is not approved of and the child learns to identify its behaviour as separate from that of the mother. Shame is present in every living human therefore. The only difference between us are the levels of shame and the ages at which they occurred developmentally. Shame and trauma are highly linked.

Traumatisation is the failure of the adaptive processing system that allows you to make sense of your experience, and crucially, for learning to take place. There is a small window of opportunity after a shameful experience for someone (usually your mother) to comfort you in a way that brings your social engagement system into play, down-regulating the more primitive fight, flight and freeze. Children can be taught this by enlightened, compassionate parenting and will show more empathy to others as a result. In the normal course of events we can then process our experience via dreams, creativity, talking with others whom we trust. When the system is sensitised by the stress response however, these processes become coded with a survival tag (in the hippocampus - the context stamp area) which makes them unavailable to normal processing. They become 'stuck' in the limbic system as intrusive thoughts, flashbacks, negative beliefs and strange body sensations which, because the memories are unconscious, can be triggered by things we have no awareness of and are powerless to change. It is a profound failure of information processing – specifically memory consolidation.

So, to summarise, trauma is anything that the mindbody finds threatening to the sense of self / survival. It can be an event that happened or one that is imagined or told to us (vicarious trauma) - such is the power of the human mind. So it is in the *interpretation and meaning* that we attribute to the event, not the event itself, that is traumatic which is why trauma is far more widespread than we first thought. I find the term 'unresolved emotion' for this helps to include more people and de-stigmatise the experience. Strictly speaking one should talk about unresolved emotional memory. Most people understand that they have unresolved emotion even if they are not willing to accept having had trauma[1]. The unfortunate result is that these past experiences colour our future experiences in unforeseen ways, as they link into our unconscious belief systems formed around the time of the trauma.

Beliefs as the filter of experience

Your beliefs about yourself and the world around you are your perceptual filter on the world. In **neuro linguistic programming (NLP)** terms they are your 'map of the world' and they profoundly affect many aspects in your life:

- Self-esteem
- Physical Health
- Relationships
- Financial prosperity
- Job security
- Spiritual connection

These messages are ultimately downloaded in childhood from the messages you were given and help to form your personality structure. Indeed most of your personality is set by the age of 7[65]. Ultimately, personality itself is an adaptation, "a way of getting out of childhood alive66" . We learn how to deal with the environment around us by developing psychic defenses (i.e. keeping our psyche intact) and behavioural traits that begin to become habitual; they are our 'coping strategies'. These may have been adaptive in the milieu in which they were formed but in later life can become dysfunctional[2].

Most people have some form of negative self-belief instilled in them by both direct experience and by absorbing the beliefs of those close to them. Usually this creates a filter on future experience – if you fundamentally

---

1 Many people I have asked on chronic fatigue / pain forums have denied any experience of trauma. When questioned in more detail however, most clearly have a traumatic past with a consequent negative self-belief system. I am about to research this as part of my PhD project via a questionnaire.

2 For more information on these coping styles (different personality types) and how they relate to different age groups of trauma see www.sabrinawyeneth.com

believe you are worthless, or you need to work hard to prove yourself worthy (that's my one), then everything you do will be coloured by that belief. You will choose jobs, partners, and life experiences that conform to that expectation. We unconsciously recreate our reality as a response to our inherent values and belief systems, whether that be in our jobs, relationships or addictions. And we re-enact them over and over again wondering why nothing changes.

Of course, none of this is conscious. You will have the best of intentions to change, to do things differently (I myself decided before writing this book that I would stop studying for a while but then signed up for a PhD!), but somehow willpower or conscious intention is not enough. It is far weaker than these subconscious programmes. So in order to change them we have to be prepared shine a light on the darkest parts of ourselves that we have been hiding from. There is no-one else who can do it but us and it means facing the feelings that we have been actively suppressing all these years. And that is why we often procrastinate about the *doing*. We are fine about reading the right books (maybe like this one or the ones on the reading list at the end); we will even go so far as to attend some seminars or workshops. But afterwards our unconscious programming habits will take over and we find that somehow we didn't find the time, other things became more important or we persuade ourselves we don't need to worry for one reason or another. I know, I've been there!

So, to summarise, beliefs are:

- a survival strategy – they enabled us to survive by keeping us safe in childhood.
- life limiting – where once they were appropriate they can become dysfunctional and programme our responses preventing us from achieving what we want in adult life
- unconscious - we have lost the ability to realise that they are separate from us, we are not in control of our habitual responses to old childhood wounds.
- habitual - they are ingrained patterns of behaviour(responses) to certain triggers.

What is trauma?

Trauma is not necessarily a major event although those are important of course. Bereavement is one such 'big T' trauma. The loss of someone we love is a profound experience which cannot be adequately expressed with words and thus is coded in implicit memory as a 'sense feeling'. Whenever that gets triggered again in later life (e.g. we lose a relationship, job or something that has meaning for us), it is ready to be brought out of memory as a feeling of sadness, loss, even though the current event may not have the same degree of loss. If the emotion is the same then the brain interprets that as a threat to survival and the limbic system is engaged. The hippocampus brings out of storage all the previous examples of that feeling and the cumulative effect of this is to re-experience all the losses at once. This explains why we can feel so easily overwhelmed because it isn't just the events currently going on that are being experienced, it is all the implicit (wordless) past memories that are being triggered and re-enacted.

However, as we are beginning to understand there are more 'everyday traumas', sometimes called 'small-t' traumas; in other words things that happen often in people's lives which in themselves are not big events but are *interpreted* as being a threat to their survival. Remember, it is not necessarily the size of the trauma but the *meaning* we ascribe to the event that counts, depending on our prior experience and sensitisation. Hence, virtually anything can be traumatic if certain factors are present; one key factor is *helplessness*.

Trauma comes about when an emotion (and the action that is supposed to be the response to that emotion) is thwarted. Peter Levine, a therapist and researcher, considers it part of the undischarged freeze response[1]. When our very selfhood is threatened, (as it is when we are unable to get help or are instead shamed into submission), it is this deeply embedded dorsal vagal system that takes over - called the 'freeze response'. If we are not able to *do something* to alleviate it, the implicit memory response is thus coded traumatically. German cancer researcher Dr Ryke Hamer calls it a 'Biological-conflict-shock'[67] involving the psyche, brain and 'organ' system.

Some common traumatic life experiences are:

- A stressful gestation (your mother experiences stress whilst carrying you) – her stress hormones are secreted into your shared blood supply
- Difficult birth (forceps delivery, premature especially if put in an incubator) – it used to be thought that babies had no way of feeling pain – we now know that is not true and they are acutely tuned in to their environment
- Poor attachment to parent – where caregiving is ambivalent, anxious or erratic
- Dentistry or surgery – especially where you are young and have no

---

1 He based this observation on studies of animals who, after they have faced a life-threatening situation, go through shaking to discharge the trauma and rebalance the Autonomic Nervous System

control
- Bullying, sibling rivalry, abuse (emotional, physical or sexual)
- Unresolved grief/ anger/ loss – especially of a significant figure e.g.a grand/ parent
- Conflicted feelings (approach /avoidance conflict, particularly with parents – you love them but you don't get what you need)
- Vicarious trauma – observing others in pain, with nothing you can do to alleviate[1]

It would be unusual to go through a childhood without one of the things on the list but the 'window of opportunity' to prevent them being encoded traumatically is very short. If, after the experience, no-one comforts you in the right way and enables you to put the experience in context (allowing the watchtower of the ACC, hippocampus and PFC to mark it as non-threatening), it is likely you will experience it as unresolved, or traumatic.I have put them in roughly chronological order because each one acts as a precursor to the next. Hence, if your earliest experiences are stressful the brain is landscaped via neuroplasticity to perceive subsequent experiences as stressful – the brain becomes wired that way. We could include in this list all manner of rejections, betrayals, humiliations and shameful feelings, some of which I described in my own childhood. You will have your own, I'm sure.

My definition of trauma therefore is broad: it is any unresolved / undischarged emotion established during a situation of helplessness. It is life limiting because it colours your perceptions and pervade everything you do.

Emotions; the language of the body

Emotions and feelings are so key to how we experience the world. They give us the depth of experience as humans but they are clearly both an advantage and, sometimes, a handicap. We must distinguish emotions from 'feelings' (sometimes called affects in psychology) which are subjective interpretations with cognitive input from the cortex. In common usage feelings and emotions are the same but neurologically, emotions are just feeling states from within the body made from neural connections. There

---

1 Remember, indirect (learnt) information can also be encoded as trauma e.g. if your parent says it's unsafe, or they react to something with fear i.e. it becomes a learned response. My mother managed to do this with me by teaching me to be afraid of spiders – although fear of crawling things is somewhat innate, you normally learn to overcome this. But if someone you grow up around has a phobia, these messages of fear are ingrained.

are 3 types:
1. Reactive: fear and defensive rage – these are primitive and hardwired[1]
2. Routine: happiness, surprise, anger, etc – learned and fleeting in prefrontal cortex
3. Reflective: require conscious thought e.g. shame, guilt, grief, jealousy, etc. Long-lived, require cognitive input and *can be traumatically encoded* in the limbic system[5].

One of the primary emotions that I deal with in any form of health challenge is fear. Fear can be motivating / enhance decision-making as it diminishes choices and helps memory retrieval in the short term. It is one of the most ancient emotions, hardwired in and conserved throughout evolution as a survival mechanism to encode fear-producing memories to avoid predation (being eaten). This takes place when the amygdala directs the hippocampus to store and retrieve encoded memories for ready retrieval in new fear-producing situations. However, we rarely have to face such primal fears these days; we have new demons to face. One of the most fear-inducing situations in life is illness (either of ourselves or others) – something that most of us have to face at some time in our life.

Becoming ill strips you of your surface 'presentation' to the world. You are no longer 'strong' and capable. Because getting ill is culturally accepted as being a weakness, this can be doubly shaming for people who have previously been highly capable and hard-working. You may suddenly be restricted in the type of work or how much you can do. As illness takes a toll on the body through having to gear up protective mechanisms it can render you without much energy or willpower to cope with it. The body's natural adaptation is to rest but this is incompatible with most people's over-busy lives and we simply refuse to allow ourselves to be ill. Internal questions over what is happening and what might happen in the future can take over our thinking. It takes a lot of strength to fight the fear which is not helped by a health service that inculcates fear at every turn through the uncertainty of tests and waiting for results. Fear is pervasive and it invades our every waking moment (and often our sleepless nights). Fear perpetuates the stress on the body and can actually slow down our recovery. Although, it may help us fight the illness, it is a double-edged sword.

There will also often be rage at being ill under the surface. Both are similar evolutionary adaptations hardwired to increase survival; rage may

---

1 Reactive and Reflective emotions are the important ones for our discussion as they do not diminish over time and produce chronic inescapable stress. As humans we have certain appetitive needs e.g. attachment, food, water and sex which promote drives which, if unmet, can also cause chronic stress

have helped us fight the predator but it is not so useful when we are ill. When the predator is yourself (through illness) or your parents (who may have hurt you) or your partner (who is dismissive or unsupportive) the rage is not so easily expressed and it becomes buried quite deeply. Even in those who can express their emotions (feelings), they are difficult to acknowledge. Because of our cultural imperatives, they are rarely openly expressed, being 'unacceptable', and an internal conflict begins whereby they are stored unconsciously because they are too frightening to the conscious mind.

This is particularly true of rage which is rarely acknowledged although it finds vent in other ways; destructive relationships, addiction to stress and drama, and often, bizarrely, overtly submissive behaviours (whilst holding huge resentment). This is never more true than in intimate relationships where to admit your needs are not being met would be too scary, so you withhold love and affection or constantly undermine the other person with subtle criticism. This is known as a passive/aggressive stance. It is very common.

Why we struggle; transforming shame

What underlies all of these 'unacceptable' feelings is *shame;* the most unacceptable emotion of all. Shame as we've seen is a normal part of growing up when it is handled well. But if it is the result of our childhood needs constantly not being met in some way, we begin to believe we are bad, wrong or somehow unacceptable[1]. In adult life we may still feel 'stupid', embarrassed, weak, vulnerable, when things are not going our way or we feel misunderstood by people. Shame shows up in ways that make us feel to blame somehow but we're not sure why. Shame is a most pervasive emotion; it not only underlies some of our most uncomfortable feelings but it pervades our culture too. Brené Brown, a US shame researcher, talks about our society constantly using the weapon of shame to make ourselves feel superior to others. Work-relationships are often shame dependent. Reality TV thrives on it. Look at women's magazines for a classic example of the end result of this never ending struggle to be 'better than' someone else.

The shame tapes that we play are many and various. These are the messages we were taught from childhood that somehow we are not worthy but the subtlety of the message is such that we don't even know that we're playing them. Here are some of the consequences:

- Excessive comparison with others, criticism and negativity

---

1 A child will create belief structures that make sense of the world as they perceive it and there is a strong survival imperative not to see their parents as being 'bad', dangerous or weak. The child will therefore make sense of the situation by making it their own fault for their inherent badness.

- Overwork, excessive drive to succeed
- Fear of failure
- Fear of success
- Perfectionism; never being good enough
- Procrastination; never being able to start or complete something (linked to the above)
- Trying to 'fit in' to a group or culture without a sense of belonging
- Rejection of relationships or acceptance of poor quality ones
- Need to be right and in control of everything
- Seeing vulnerability as a weakness

Brené Brown has studied the causes and solutions to shame-based living from a study of over 2000 adults. She says "we live in a culture where overworking and exhaustion is a status symbol and productivity is self-worth"7. Her research led her to want to find the solutions to encourage more joyful living. They are:

- self-worth & self-love
- vulnerability
- rest
- play
- creativity

The first two points are absolutely key as you cannot build loving connection with others unless you have self-love as a baseline – but it's not easy as the default is the opposite. The second is also essential as you cannot have connection with others without making yourself vulnerable – but we have strong defences against this too. The remaining ones depend on the first two and are the features of our lives we are most likely to lose as we play the 'shame-game'. We will persuade ourselves there simply isn't enough time.

These characteristics of shame-free or what Brené calls 'whole-hearted living' shocked her and caused her to review her whole life. In doing so she created a new life based around teaching these approaches. However, in doing so she came up against all the same issues that prevent us from incorporating these into our lives. Here are the blocks to change that I experienced and am now presented with often with my clients.

Blocks to Change

We have a low tolerance for frustration, and slow changes. We have been brought up to expect things to be instant and easy, even more so today in the world of instant communications. We have no frame of reference for complex emotional situations which require flexibility and openness while we learn how to engage with our own or another person's emotional landscape. Hence we use that wonderful technique of avoidance of conflict; running away, moving on, blaming the other person, etc. But we find that strangely those situations just keep coming back and life repeats itself like re-running the same play just with new characters.

Then we avoid things that trigger the same shame feelings, so we cut down our play, social contacts and creativity further. We numb with whatever our childhood pattern tells us is comforting (food, TV, etc), but the things that trigger us broaden until we find we are perpetuating rather than resolving the issue. The end result can be many forms of anxiety and depressive illness. Bizarrely, we even *re-enact* rather than resolve which is a common pattern in many people. I see many clients who, after having a childhood filled with trauma, go on to have multiple car accidents or abusive relationships. It is not that they are consciously deciding to repeat the painful situation, it is a subconscious process of re-enactment which is a defensive pattern doomed to failure as it seldom resolves the underlying issue which is one of shame.

After a while we may adopt 'learned helplessness' which is a term coined by US researcher Martin Seligman in his research on dogs who repeatedly got electric shocks and eventually failed to move out of the way. He maintains that human beings have the same response in that we lose faith that we can change and so we give up. It seems easier to stay with what we know. We can also dissociate or freeze off our emotions eventually – we are not even in touch with emotions so no longer know what messages they are telling us. This has physical health consequences; from chronic pain to heart disease, as our bodies read our (subconscious) minds.

Finally we *fear change*. Change of any sort is scary. We are creatures of habit, which includes our emotions. Even if the emotions (feelings) are uncomfortable, at least they are familiar. We dig our heels in, show '*resistance*' if anyone questions us and carry on doing what we've always done. I know in my own life, when running a business,. I am constantly comparing myself to others, which I initially experience as a wave of fear and my mind judges whether I am 'good enough' doing it my way. That will often globalise to being good enough generally i.e. at *what* I do, not *how* I do it. Most of us (and particularly women I find) are not good at believing in ourselves, we have accepted the notion that somehow we are defective, and that self-worth is dependent on what we *do* (which is a constant task) and not who we *are*. This is the essence of shame.

To counter shame then requires some work. Firstly it needs you to identify the ways in which shame shows up in your life. Are there things you avoid, things you do to numb yourself, self-explanations of how things are that allow you to forever put off challenging yourself or owning what is in your heart? It is easier if you have someone around you who is willing to be present when you speak of these things and not talk down to you, tell you it's not so bad and to get on with it, or otherwise devalues your experience. There is a vast difference between those who show you sympathy ('oh poor you, it must be really bad in that hole') and empathy ('oh yes me too, let me come down with you and we'll work it out'). It takes guts for people to really hear your shame because they have their own and talking about yours triggers them. That's why it is so infernally difficult. It requires willingness and patience to hear another's story without wanting to:

- fix it
- have more stories than they have (oneupmanship)
- dismiss it

So choose the person to work through your shame with wisely; someone who has dealt with their own and understands the difficulty it entails as well as the resistance that is likely to come up. The rewards though are worth it; health, abundance and joy in life, the resilience to show up and be present not just despite what is happening but because of it. I know because this is what I had to do to get well. Owning the fact that I was miserable because I felt unloved was one of the biggest challenges to me. I had always been the strong one so admitting to weakness and vulnerability was huge. I encourage you to prioritise your emotional health equally to your physical. As we have seen they are not separate, and both are vital if you want to live fully and well.

Chapter 7: The Body Speaks the Mind; Trauma and Chronic Disease

As we have seen, up until recently we have had a medical model constructed on the separateness of mind and body. Hence a physical pain or problem is understood to have a physical cause and mental illness is 'in your head' or 'psychosomatic'. This is a profoundly limiting and potentially dangerous dogma that has considerable consequences for the health of our population. However, more recently, beginning with the investigations into PNI in the 1990's, there has been considerable interest in the idea of *emotions* as an important contributor to physical pain. One of the main contributors in the field of chronic pain was Dr John Sarno, Professor of Rehabilitation Medicine in the US and, until his retirement in 2012, an attending physician in a rehabilitation centre. He began to be interested in his patients' mental/emotional experience of the pain and what he discovered became a ground-breaking new theory which has been subsequently developed by James Alexander and others.

Central nervous system sensitisation - brain pain

So, with our model of the mind as consisting of both front (cortical) and back (limbic and brainstem) brains we can see that the brain has separate pathways for making sense of the world. At the moment of trauma the brain has a decision to make. Incoming information from the senses are relayed by an area called the thalamus (think of it as the 'cook' (mixing incoming signals) and gatekeeper (it directs attention to what needs to be focussed on within the 'autobiographical soup'). The thalamus makes a judgement as to whether the information is sufficiently threatening as to need to go the 'High Road' (front brain) or the 'Low Road' (back brain) which is much faster[68].

Figure 23 Sensory Pathways of the Brain

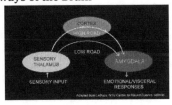

The high road is slower because it involves a lot more complex cortical processing. The low road is our survival brain with a lot of involuntary, automatic functions which allow the alarm (amygdala) to be sounded if the input is deemed to be threatening enough. When that happens, as we've seen, the HPA axis is fired using the sympathetic nervous system and the whole cycle of nerve and hormone signals is set into motion with potentially devastating consequences.

Normally, if this thwarts the trauma threat the system re-sets and normality resumes. However, with repeated trauma the low road becomes the default pathway as the amygdala becomes sensitised. The high road is diverted, and every potential threat is seen by the amygdala as a real one so that even ambiguous or uncertain situations trigger the response. Indeed even the fear of a threat occurring is enough to trigger it; this is what happens in panic attacks when the body detects its own **interoceptive** signals (increasing heart rate etc) as a threat. We become wired for fear. Recovery is about interrupting these habitual signals and rerouting back to the high road where the cortex and hippocampus can properly evaluate and add context. Unfortunately for most people they (and their healthcare practitioners) have no idea this is going on and the symptoms themselves become fear-inducing. When you worry that your health is in decline and there's nothing you can do you further exacerbate the problem. Our central brain systems are set 'high' for pain sensitivity and we react to perceived threat by the default stress pathway. We are then set up for chronic disease and pain.

An epidemic of mindbody disease; chronic pain and fatigue-related syndromes

It seems incredible to think given all that we now know, that modern medicine should still have so little understanding of the mindbody link in chronic pain and chronic fatigue related syndromes (CRFS) like Fibromyalgia and Chronic Fatigue. It leaves a huge number of people suffering without hope or help.

Initially perhaps, it does seem paradoxical that chronic pain could result from something that goes on in our brains but as we have seen there are many pathways that directly influence our physiology. There are two reasons why this is so important with chronic pain. Firstly, pain is a *subjective experience*. There is no sensory 'pain' organ. There are organs that tell us about stretch and rupture, for instance if we sprain our ankle, we feel pain. But the signals that are sent to the brain are not inherently pain signals. Pain then is constructed; with an emotional component created in the brain from various signals the brain receives, both from the damaged parts of the body and other parts of brain which help 'code' or interpret the signals. If you doubt this think about when you've cut yourself and it doesn't hurt till you suddenly notice it – or when soldiers are injured in battle they often feel nothing at first. Plus, if it means that they can now go home and are out of the war they often feel euphoria, not pain. It is the subjective *meaning* of the pain that is able to alter the experience.

Secondly, the way that the brain interprets pain shares pathways with other sensations and the brain does its best to make sense of the incoming signals. Our brain's complexity is such that emotional pain shares a lot of the same neural pathways with physical pain. In particular, brain researchers have found, it shares pathways with 'centres that record social ruptures and rejection'[69]. So, if you've had a loss in your life whether it be a person or an identity or your health for instance, your body often expresses this loss in physical pain. It's something that astounded me when I first discovered this but its truth has been proven to me over and over again as I assess clients' pain and find the same patterns returning. The brain creates pain in specific ways with an overlay of emotions and cognitions (thoughts about the pain). The pain can vary in whether it is **nocioceptive** (due to tissue damage), **neuropathic** (due to nerve damage), or **psychogenic** – the latter is defined by the absence of an identifiable physical cause i.e. it is a learned pain response rather than pathological.

There are certain patterns to the pain that occur in people despite their differing makeup.

Back pain is often a feature of repressed anger or a deep sense of internal conflict (e.g. experiencing severe difficulties in a job but you cannot quit[70]), shoulders usually express a burden of over-responsibility, knees and legs a fear of moving forward. I know this sounds like cloud cuckoo land to some of you – it did to me but it seems in terms of the neural pathways all emotions are not the same and they are coded in specific parts of the mindbody. The location of pain on the left and right sides also seem to be important; left is considered to relate to mother and right to father. Louise Hay detailed more of the typical patterns in her book 'Heal your Life'[71]). Before you dismiss this have a look at her descriptions and see if you can recognise any correlation in your pain.

In addition to the specific pain patterns, there is a general overall amplification of pain in most individuals with chronic pain. Dr. Dan Clauw, the Director of the Chronic Pain & Fatigue Center at the University of Michigan, likens it to an electric guitar (the sensory nerves in the periphery) playing the same tune but the amplifier (central nervous system - CNS) amplifying the signal inappropriately. The CNS has an important role in modulating pain messages from the body; when operating correctly it should be able to inhibit pain interpretation in the brain from non-painful stimuli. When this is not functioning well, the inhibition is absent and virtually anything e.g. sitting in a chair or being touched becomes painful.

The amplifier is simply turned up too high. I believe this **allodynia** is a stress response, related to unprocessed emotions which have set the body on high alert. Here is a diagram that shows the journey from the pain stimulus (1) being received by a nocioceptor (noxious stimulus receptor) in the periphery up the sensory nerve fibres (purple – fast alpha fibres and black slower unmyelinated fibres which travel to the spinal cord (shown in section) then up to specific parts of the brain (3). But the important part to note is (2) the green fibres of modulatory **interneurons** from the midbrain which inhibit the pain pathway. If these are not functioning more pain is felt i.e. amplified.

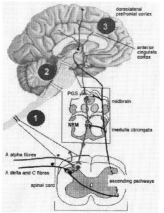

Figure 24 The pain pathways

When I trained in Emotional Freedom Technique (EFT- described in more detail in the last chapter) one of the other students was a lady who had chronic knee pain. She had had innumerable visits to consultants and doctors with no real benefit. We did two days of training and then on the final day, when she had got comfortable with the process, the trainer decided to use her as a case study to demonstrate on and she valiantly came forward. He went through the tapping procedure (there is a sequence of 'points' on the head and neck) whilst she stated the affirmation (the so-called 'set-up phrase') which was something like: 'even though I have this aching knee pain I deeply and completely accept myself anyway'. This was repeated as she reported any thoughts or feelings that popped up whilst doing the tapping. These associations are very common in **psychosensory therapies** (described in chapter 8) and are controlled by the limbic system having made connections between certain events in your past where the same emotion was evoked. The brain is a pattern-matching organ and it is hard-wired for survival so that events which are frightening or threatening will be coded permanently for future avoidance.

After 2 or 3 repetitions of the tapping procedure, on each feeling/ association she was asked to stand up and see how her knee felt. This woman had assessed her pain initially as an 8 or 9 on a 10 point scale and she was absolutely shocked that when she stood up the pain had dropped to a 4 or 5! No-one was more surprised than me. I had heard EFT was good for anxiety, cravings and addictions i.e. *mental* issues. I had never seen it used on physical pain before. At that time I had no idea what mechanism could explain this astounding result, now I know that her unprocessed feelings were activating certain nerves.

Careful questioning by the trainer elucidated that the pain had come on not long after her father's death. It wasn't hard to make the connection between that loss and her current knee pain – he could have left it at that but cleverly he decided to look at barriers to losing the pain. She clearly had been devastated by his loss and had no idea what to do with her life without him. But there was also a part of her that wanted to keep the pain as it was preferable to dealing with his loss and this was the part that the trainer then worked on. This was so that she could let go of her pain but keep her memory of her father. Somehow these two had been conflated in her mind, and once she could really grieve for him, the pain no longer had a function. Over several subsequent sessions, she was able to release it and she could now move on – both figuratively and physically. She ended the three days with hardly any pain at all which was a revelation to her and the beginning of understanding of mindbody connections for me.

Sometimes, the mindbody holds on to pain in preference to dealing with the real issue of emotional pain; the unconscious may make the mistaken assumption that giving up the pain is somehow a *betrayal* of the person that you are holding it for. The limbic system's role is to keep us safe but the traumatic memory encoding sometimes has the opposite effect and may serve to keep us stuck in old patterns of behaving and feeling – running a program that may have saved us when we were little but is ill-suited to our current life. The physical results are many and various and this book can't possibly cover them all. For a more detailed look at the auto-immune disorders for instance (Rheumatoid Arthritis, Lupus, Crohn's Disease, Sjogren's etc) I refer you to other books[72] on that complex subject area. I will restrict myself to those issues I see regularly in my clinic; the more common manifestations of these 'medically unexplained symptoms' (MUS – or various 'medically unexplained syndromes'[1]) starting with the most common.

Chronic fatigue Syndrome (CFS)

Chronic fatigue, or 'yuppie flu' as it was once known, began to be recognised on a large scale during the 1990's. At first doctors were baffled when people began complaining of unremitting fatigue not relieved by rest, insomnia and pain. Sufferers would generally be considered depressed and told to go home and rest, or worse still they were told it was all in their mind and to get on with it. The terrible legacy of that ignorance is that even now, 25 years later, medical students still have to be taught that it is a *real* disease[1].

← • It has a remarkable gender differential with more than 7/10 sufferers being women. There are various theories why this is so:

- Testosterone prevents adrenal fatigue (one of the initiating factors).

- Men have less hormonal fluctuation and are thus less likely to get out of balance.

- Women may be more prone to freeze (parasympathetic dominance) than fight or flight (sympathetic dominance) – a genetic difference?

Women tend to have more concomitant conditions with it – so called 'co-morbidity' - and these map to a higher prevalence of auto-immune and depressive complaints generally. Whilst researchers debate these differences, few outside the psychiatric profession have made the physical link with trauma. Because they don't understand the physical nature of many of these unconscious effects it is often dismissed as a diversion to the discovery of the real *physical* cause. Many patient and support groups have made the link however.

According to the Chrysalis Effect and the Optimum Health Clinic, both organisations that have pioneered recovery from CFS, it is a multifactorial disease with strong psychological drivers. It has been noted that it often affects high achieving people who are highly motivated, driven, and often in denial of their own needs i.e. people-pleasing. There is no doubt that the personality factors are equally important as the physical.

Many people with the condition believe it is viral, or at the very least

---

1 Syndromes are conditions of unknown origin whose diagnoses are based on a collection of typical symptoms that therefore characterise the illness.

1 I have been present at recent lectures at my university where visiting scholars spend the first half-an-hour persuading their sceptical audience of the fact that it is a real disease and not made up.

they can link it to a viral infection – like Epstein Barr for instance. Most will have an event which tipped them over the edge and which they believe 'caused' the illness. Our current understanding though is that this is merely the 'straw that broke the camel's back' and in fact, you need the other drivers in place for the condition to develop. Most likely these were in place from childhood onwards. Work by Dr. Sarah Myhill and others has uncovered much of the basic biochemical imbalances, particularly in the mitochondria which underlie these conditions[73].

They maintain that chronic fatigue is a problem of mitochondrial dysfunction (mitochondriopathy), which I would agree with. We have already described how the mitochondria are able to sense environmental issues of low oxygen and stress which divert the metabolism into low energy production (glycolysis or fermentation). The problem still remains that we are uncertain what causes the cell to sense danger and go into the go-slow pathway.

It clearly has physical determinants; toxicity (and the overwhelm of the detoxification systems), nutrient deficiency (lack of co-factors required for the chemical reactions of the cell), etc which all seem to play their part. Certainly, changing your diet is the first step in recovery. But attending to the purely physical seems to only get you so far and it begs the question 'why did the body sense danger – what are the signals that enable it to get so run down?' The answer in my view is unprocessed trauma or emotionally encoded memories.

Trauma as the signal for mitochondrial dysfunction

My own observation has been that trauma seems to be a common factor in many sufferers' personal histories[1]. Because these traumas may not be conscious, or they are of the cumulative or 'small-t' type, they may not have been recognised as contributing factors in development of the disease. Doctors (and even psychiatrists sadly) are not trained to look and seldom ask about trauma. In any case not everyone who suffers from the symptoms has a firm diagnosis, they may not have developed sufficient symptoms to warrant treatment or even a trip to the doctor so the links have not been made. People are very resistant to the idea of a disease that has a link with mental health and thus there is much stigma and misunderstanding around it. They may manage with the symptoms for a long time before 'the crash' phase where their usual coping mechanisms finally give way. According to the Chrysalis Effect, there are usually typical 'Early warning signs[74]' that

---

1 My PhD, ongoing at the time of writing, is looking at this very question

occur before the onset of full symptoms. These include;
Early Warning Signs of Chronic Fatigue style syndromes
- Anxiety, restlessness
- Insomnia, waking early or difficulty staying asleep
- Headaches/Migraines
- Intolerance to alcohol, gut problems (IBS)
- Pins and needles, strange body sensations
- Poor concentration, fuzzy headed feeling
- Sensitivity to noise, or other stimulation
- Dizziness (vertigo)

They are all signs that something in the body is out of balance, and it is likely we will ignore them at first, putting it down to normal 'stress' (whatever that is). We adopt certain adaptations to our lifestyle to cope. These coping mechanisms include:
- Living on caffeine, energy drinks and sugary foods to get you through the day
- Having to sleep most of the weekend to keep up with your weekly schedule
- Cutting down on those things that make you happy i.e. your social life in order to keep working
- Increasing alcohol (to help you 'relax')
- Going to bed early to be able to cope with work
- Starting a gym routine to 'build stamina'
- Taking sleeping tablets and anti-depressants to keep you going

I had a lot of these symptoms when I first got ill and my solution was pretty much this too. It is normal to be in denial because of fear that something is terribly wrong with you (we all have a tendency to imagine the worst). In actual fact, there *is* something very wrong but it is nothing to fear; it is something that needs addressing and facing however. The precursors of chronic fatigue or auto-immune disease may start with these symptoms but if ignored are only likely to get worse as the stress of illness takes its toll. Note that it is the particular *combination* of contributing events (usually early trauma and gut imbalance which affects nutrient levels and metabolic function) that cumulatively combines to weaken the body until there is a 'tipping point' at which the body goes into outright exhaustion. This is the 'crash' that many people report as the beginning of their illness.

It may be triggered by an infection, a death, emotional conflict, or accident, but the precursors were there many years before, it just needed all factors in place to become CFS/ Auto-Immune Disease or whatever.

It seems to affect predominantly women, although men and children are affected, and is a growing problem – estimates are that it affects approximately 2.54% of the population[75]. In the UK the ME Association calculates 254,000 people are currently suffering from ME/CFS although I suspect if you included people who are not yet diagnosed or who are showing first symptoms it is probably a lot higher. Because of the history of controversy around the disease and the emotional/ personality factors that help drive it, it just doesn't 'fit' within the current paradigm of Western medicine so is very poorly managed. But we have to look at it as a 'biopsychosocial' illness with inputs from all three areas and this enables us to treat it effectively. When you are in emotional denial of your own needs and yet driven to prove yourself in a world that constantly undermines or ignores you, it is not surprising that illness results. It just seems that this imbalance is increasing, and it seems to fall particularly on females, people in the 'years of responsibility', and the young in that order. Stress is obviously a big factor but of course how we interpret stress depends on our biology, our psychology and how society relates to us. You can see it is a complex picture.

Death by speciality; how modern medicine fails to see the bigger picture

Modern medicine (and psychiatry which is the mental offshoot) do some things extremely well. In fact it is a miracle when it comes to solving acute problems that would have once killed you. Antibiotics are a classic example of scientific innovation from the last century that have saved countless lives. Recent innovations in drug delivery and nano medicine are making huge inroads into what were once debilitating conditions. Surgical expertise and acute care makes survival into old age much more likely. My mother who is in her 80's recently had a pacemaker fitted and it was done under local anaesthetic with an overnight stay. That would have once been an extremely serious operation that would have entailed a long recovery. That is incredible and will probably extend her life by many years. In the UK where we have the National Health Service (NHS) this is paid for by national insurance and so is free at the point of need. How amazing... I am extremely grateful and honour the men and women who are at the heart of our health service. They work so hard under increasing workloads and often bear the brunt of political expediency and a blame culture.

However, where problems are of a chronic, long-term nature and the issues are compounded with psychological factors, there is a greater chance that modern medicine will fail you. It has been said that "there is a profound disconnect between scientific evidence and medical practice"[76]. We are still looking at disease within the biomedical frame based on an infectious disease model, treating symptoms as if they were the cause as we do with infection; by applying this approach to disease such as CFS we end up treating the fever instead of the bacterium, so to speak. Firstly, if you get diagnosed at all (it make take years and you may be accused of malingering), your GP may have very little to offer you beside painkillers and anti-depressants. You then get sent from specialist to specialist who each have their own viewpoint and treatment routines which don't necessarily join up with what you have been told before leading to confusion and an endless round of tests, results and medications. When all this has been exhausted you may still not have any coherent plan for recovery and end up doubting your own reality, which further stresses you. Finally they may wash their hands of you as they no longer know what to do to help you.

The essential problem is modern medicine has tied itself to the mast of pharmaceutical and surgical intervention. Medical education is largely funded by pharmaceutical companies and its large corporations dictate what is taught. You might not believe me here but if you follow the history from President Roosevelt's administration onwards you will find that 'Big Pharma', as it is affectionately known, was hugely influential in changing the nature of medical teaching back in the 1930's away from 'folk remedies' (i.e. natural medicine) and what they regarded as 'quackery' and towards the new, modern solution.

Where America led, the rest of the developed world has largely followed. We threw the baby out with the bathwater. We lost some unproven and dangerous practices but we also lost some very important information on nutrition, herbal medicine and mindbody approaches which was largely forgotten. Today, you either go 'mainstream' with the pharma/surgical approach or you go private and alternative if you want to explore other approaches. There is not only little cross-fertilisation but there is also active derision from the powerful mainstream towards less well-funded but nevertheless effective treatments.

In confusion, people end up trying to find their own solutions which results in a very ad-hoc/ 'pick n mix' approach which is dependent on their consultant or therapist's understanding of the underlying factors. Unfortunately this varies as much in the alternative world as it does in the mainstream.

There is the complicating factor that some practitioners are wedded to the idea that something is either physical or mental/emotional – their training may fail to thoroughly teach the integrated view (both conventional and alternative). Some physical therapists (in or outside the mainstream), for instance, may actually make the chronic pain client inadvertently worse as they help to support the view that there is a structural cause for the pain which means the client continues to wait for the magic solution and avoids looking at some of the less obvious internally-generated triggers. This keeps therapists and consultants in business but it does not always provide a solution to the client. It was this factor that prompted me to start learning more about the mind as I was not getting the results for my clients with a purely physical approach. In addition, the placebo factor of being state supported ('white coat effect'), which is what actually helps people to heal more effectively than some drugs and surgery, has not been available to those of us who operate outside of the state-funded health service[1]. I would love to be state supported and licensed but, in the UK, unlike the US and some European countries, neither massage nor hypnotherapy is recognised. It is a sad state of affairs which means unless we elevate ourselves by serious research and advertising we end up being dismissed as 'quacks' peddling 'flakey' therapies.

When I first was setting up my therapy business I was advised NOT to call myself a 'holistic' therapist because 'nobody would take me seriously'[2]. Unfortunately the word holistic has been taken up by the new age movement with an assortment of unproven therapies which are the subject of much ridicule in the popular press and online[3]. Sadly its true origins in (w)holism, health and healing[4] have been forgotten. This is unfortunate. The holistic model offers much that is extremely valuable; it takes the person first and the issue/problem second. In other words when you go and see a person who offers holistic (integrated) medicine they are more interested in the person with the illness than the illness a person has. This is a completely different way of viewing health.

We take as a starting point that not all illnesses with the same name have the same causes in all people. Every person is unique and their particular

---

1 Therapists who are state-sanctioned may benefit by engendering a positive expectation of success in their clients. When someone walks into a clinic that has a certain cachet attached, the clients invariably do better because they may believe in the power of the consultant/therapist.

2 Another hypnotherapist in my professional support group said this to me.

3 I have received scathing attacks online by 'internet trolls', for daring to suggest that homoeopathy may work vibrationally (i.e a quantum effect) rather than chemically. I retain on open mind on things I don't understand but not everyone does. Be aware if you step outside the mainstream that there are vested interests at work to deride and denigrate your efforts.

4 They share the same derivation.

drivers for illness will be different. Labelling all people as their illness is simply not helpful in this paradigm. As we are not going to be prescribing the same thing for each condition, it is unnecessary. Using a functional approach to medicine is radically different – we look at the underlying condition of the mindbody; its detoxification pathways, nutritional and psychological health. When these are looked at we often see a unique pattern of sub-optimal functioning which may not show up in hospital/clinic tests (which can only find serious dysfunction outside normal population ranges) but nevertheless have serious consequences for you. And, as we have seen, one of the main causes, mitochondrial dysfunction, is not routinely tested for at all! A functional approach looks at you as the sum total of your biochemistry, genetics and life experience and seeks to piece together what is happening and why. It does not tie itself to the diagnosis in the same way but instead looks at the true causes[1].

At the heart of all my therapy and indeed the writing of this book is the wish to show you, as I do my clients, that by understanding how this process works you can understand your illness, pain or other symptoms, not as *being* you but as a function of your mindbody[2]. Gaining this distance between what you perceive and what you *are* (interrupting the identification with your illness i.e. 'I am a chronic pain sufferer') enables you to develop compassion for yourself, and others, that allows you to release the judgement and break the anxiety cycle which contributes to more pain and dysfunction. Ultimately, you allow yourself to grow spiritually and experience joy and love *even with the problem* until finally you are able to heal. Without this mindfulness, you are stuck identifying with your pain, and your anxiety and disconnect continue to grow.

Healing Chronic Pain and Fatigue syndromes

The 'management' of pain in the current medical model is one of powerlessness and continual pharmaceutical/surgical intervention which keep you subject to the decisions of the 'experts' and in a whirlpool of worry and fear, not to mention repeated trauma. This is indeed a spiritual no-man's land. It's no wonder that many people suffer for decades. True healing comes about when we are able to really connect with ourselves and listen to our bodies in ways which we have steadfastly denied[3]. It is not

---

1 Some clients search for a diagnosis as if it was the Holy Grail. They believe that once they have the 'correct' one then the cure will thus be found. Unfortunately, chronic conditions often defy diagnosis or a diagnosis is in itself only descriptive and not diagnostic e.g.fibromyalgia.

2 Pain itself is formed in the brain by interpreting neural signals and is subject to bias, emotional overlay and interpretation. It is not a subjective experience via 'pain' neurons.

about finding the 'right' approach as many different approaches can work for different people. If you find yourself getting frustrated or upset because you are not getting better as quickly as you expected, and move on to the next thing and the next, you will only delay your recovery. Tuning into yourself and recognising your psychological pattern of having to 'fix it' is the key here which some have called 'living life without resistance'[77].

The first aim of my approach is to allow people to accept where they are and to stop the struggle. It is a curious fact that the more you fight against something the more it comes back at you – particularly where emotions are involved. This does not mean 'giving in' – far from it. Acceptance means coming to terms with the situation as it is now but from a place of peace and understanding instead of fear. Many people misunderstand this idea; indeed they live their entire lives struggling against their imperfections. They believe that once they have certain things in place, they will be happy, whether it is the right person, the right job or the removal of pain. Making a fundamental decision to be happy *whatever* your circumstance is the first aim of this acceptance approach and has even been embraced by the mainstream in pain management[78]. In essence, we are trying to counter hopelessness which is both the beginning and the continuation of trauma as we have seen and further exacerbates whatever pain or health issues you have. Vaclav Havel once said *"Hope is an orientation of the spirit, an orientation of the heart. It is not the conviction that something will turn out well, but the certainty that something makes sense regardless of how it turns out."*[79] That is the orientation therapists such as myself are hoping to turn you to.

Of course, this may sound glib when you are in the worst throes of an illness, particularly if it involves chronic pain or fatigue. Pain is a very intensely unpleasant experience which can colour every other experience and make day to day living very hard work. But getting to grips with the meaning of your pain is so important and this is where finding emotional balance comes in. Finding ways to let go of the internal battle and be still where you are is not only helpful in terms of reducing your overall experience of pain but it is absolutely vital in your eventual recovery.

A lot has been written about this in many areas of mindfulness training but a book which is especially relevant to trauma and emotional recovery is Mindsight by Daniel Siegel. He gives practical ways in which you can re-

---

3 Healing does not necessarily mean curing. Sometimes we can reduce the pain, or help people to manage it better. Ideally we would aim to remove the pain or heal the condition but sometimes this is not possible if it is too ingrained. Our main aim is to be able to remove the fear and maximise healing potential, usually the mindbody can then regain lost function to some extent.

train your mind to reduce pain and anguish. In the area of chronic pain there are only a few books which cover the mindbody approach. One I would recommend is by James Alexander, an Australian psychotherapist[57]. He describes very fully how physical pain may come about from mental/emotional causes. His basic premise, developed on from Dr John Sarno's work, is that the brain under threat sends signals to the heart to reduce the blood supply to muscles and nerves, which causes hypoxia (lack of oxygen). This then affects their functioning (from mitochondrial energy production failure). With muscles you may get cramping, weakness, and ongoing pain, especially when touched, but often also at rest. When the nerves are involved the sensation of pain may be even more acute (as nerves are more sensitive to lack of oxygen) and you may also get tingling or odd prickling sensations as well as excruciating pain. I have also encountered ticklishness in people which I believe is a lesser version of this oxygen deprivation-stimulated altered sensation – a form of body dissociation.

The range of symptoms is as vast as the human capacity to feel but the pain pattern tends to be in specific areas. The postural muscles are usually the first affected; those of the shoulder, back and pelvis. These are the hardest working muscles as they are in use even when we are at rest – again if mitochondrial dysfunction is at the heart then the energy requirement of these muscles will be especially high and not fulfilled. This would also explain why we get problems with dizziness and brain fog in these conditions – the heart and brain have the highest energy requirements of the body and thus if your mitochondria are failing these organs will be most affected.

In conventional medicine as we will see in some of the case studies, the pain will be attributed to specific injury in or around the area of pain. Scans of the affected part seem to confirm the problem – particularly with back pain. Obviously if you have back pain the problem must be in the back, right? Not necessarily.

Let's be clear – there are occasions when this is so. Cancer pain, for instance, is absolutely not to be ignored as it is a sign that tissue damage is occurring. Also, if you have an acute injury of the back then you may well have strained a ligament or have an impingement on a nerve fibre by an inflamed muscle or extruded disk. But such acute injuries are usually fully healed within three months or so and the pain gradually reduces, especially when rested. These are termed *acute* injuries. However, in chronic or now more correctly called **persistent pain** of more than three months duration we start to see a different pattern emerging; the pain does not diminish but will tend to increase or vary in intensity for reasons which seem unconnected to exercise. Rest does not seem to make much difference and often the pain is worst at night. This is a chronic pain syndrome of which whiplash is a classic example. Long after the muscles, tendons, etc have healed the pain with its tenderness, headaches and anxiety remains.

There is a whole insurance industry based on these chronic injuries (as was the case with RSI back in the 1990's) so people become convinced of their seriousness and long-term effects. Whiplash is an absolutely classic example of trauma – you are helpless in a car when you are rear-ended (usually, some people may experience it after a sideways collision). The sensations you have at the time of the accident are stored in procedural memory as sudden movement and fear. If you are then immobilised afterwards (which often happens either because you are stuck or because you are told to keep still for protection of the neck), your body is unable to complete a protective motion like running away, etc. In animals shaking would naturally be seen after such an event, which would help dissipate the trapped energy and resolve the procedural memory, but we tend to dissuade people from such overt signs of shock. We are expected to go home, rest and get over it. However, the body remembers and keeps the memory stored for you in order to help you avoid a future situation but unfortunately this then associates with any situation in which you feel helpless (and it may scare you enough to stop driving for a while). Add to this the fear and worry over loss of income, etc and you have the classic drivers for whiplash syndrome.

What makes the pain of these chronic syndromes so different is that they often get worse with time, and particularly after periods of stress. I see a lot of chronic pain in my clinic and I can usually also do a quick test to see whether we are dealing with emotionally driven pain (John Sarno calls it **Tension Myoneural Syndrome or TMS**) by taking someone through a few rounds of tapping (an EFT routine – see later). If the pain moves or is in some way changed by this procedure then I know we are dealing with a psychosomatic issue. This is not to say the pain isn't real of course. Sadly this term has been grossly misused and misunderstood by the mainstream media. We are talking about a physical end result, just that the cause is emotionally driven.

The picture is very complex and difficult to diagnose, even with the plethora of tests now available to most GPs. Tests are not always as reliable an indicator as modern medicine would have you believe. The issue comes down to the standardisation of the results into 'normal' ranges which are statistical upper and lower limits *designed by looking at populations* not individuals. Hence your results can come out 'normal' with regard to these ranges but in fact your function is far from optimal. I refer you to some of the excellent books on the subject (see in the reference section) which show you how to interpret the results of such tests and get yourself back to health. Don't take your doctor's word for it – they may not have all the information you need. They are not experts and seldom know about nutritional interventions, being much more likely to put you on synthetic hormones or drugs of one sort or another. Testing is also at the heart of nutritional therapy (a form of therapy that uses food as medicine). But here the tests are likely to be much more sensitive specific, and less geared towards outright malfunction[1].

The Adrenal/ thyroid connection

Very commonly with any sort of Chronic fatigue related syndrome (CRFS), adrenal function will be poor because of the constant stress. Cortisol, which is the main long-term stress hormone, is initially constantly pumped out by the adrenal glands and is therefore in excess, but after a while even that adaptation begins to wear out and you are more likely to have low cortisol levels, particularly in the morning when you need it to kick start you into action.

Figure 25

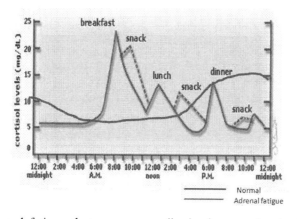

Circadian rhythm and your cortisol cycle

With adrenal fatigue that necessary spike in the morning is absent and instead you flatline in the morning which makes it difficult to get up. Then, during the day the levels slowly rise and actually peak later in the evening

---

1 Take the example of thyroid function where GPs' test ranges are only looking for Grave's disease (extreme hypthyroidsim) or Hashimoto's thyroiditis (extreme hyperthyroidism). Most people will fall somewhere in between. They don't even recognise adrenal fatigue as a real condition!

when fatigue sufferers often feel the best they have all day. This then makes it difficult for them to go to bed and rest because they are 'making up for lost time'! 'Adrenal fatigue' as it is called has many symptoms (some of which are shared with the low thyroid condition) including:

- Adrenal Fatigue symptoms
- Brain fog, cloudy-headedness and mild depression
- Low thyroid function
- Blood sugar imbalances, such as hypoglycemia
- Fatigue – especially morning and mid-afternoon fatigue
- Sleep disruption
- Low blood pressure
- Lowered immune function
- Inflammation

Note that once the adrenal function is poor, then the thyroid is also likely to be affected. Hence it is very likely both will be below par. It is very important that you get specialist help when trying to rebalance these important hormone levels because trying to treat the thyroid without first addressing the adrenals is like trying to pump the gas without the car in gear. It can overload the system and actually cause more stress and thus trigger the adrenals to make you feel *worse*[80]. Unfortunately this is what happens quite frequently with conventional or 'ad-hoc' approaches. You need someone who understands the syndrome, who is able to do tests and /or measurements of your function (and most GPs deny it exists) and can tailor it specifically to your metabolism. A nutritional therapist who specialises in this would be best, but I refer you particularly to the various books by Drs Michael Lam and James Wilson[81,82] if you want to learn more.

You will find a lot of information on the internet about supplements and home testing kits and so on. Be careful and do try to consult a naturopath or nutritional therapist at least once to get professional advice. You can do more harm than good by trying it out without sufficient knowledge. Also be aware that the same companies that are trying to sell your their expensive products will seldom tell you about the subconscious stress trigger that needs to be tackled alongside the nutritional. There are vague references to 'stress' as a causative factor but interestingly the whole alternative health field relies on it to sell their products. It can actually stress you out to feel that you need to find the answer for yourself and you feel fearful that you don't know enough. You will often find people running from one 'magic solution' to the next with little clue that what is running the show is their own anxiety. My one recommendation is get clear of your anxiety first, before you start loading your body with supplements. Just knowing that you can work slowly towards a goal lets your body know that you are in a process of healing not a quick fix situation with all the attendant stress of making mistakes. The stress factor is the one that I tackle first before getting into the specifics. Unresolved emotions take a lot of energy to keep going and because they keep you on high alert physiologically undermine your efforts to improve your physical health.

The emotion connection

The unconscious (hidden) stress of the negative emotions you harbour is like a constant flame under a pot of boiling water. The Chrysalis Effect describes it as the 'full emotional cup' of different stress factors which eventually spills over[83].

Figure 26 The Emotional Cup (thanks to Liz Dyde)

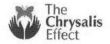

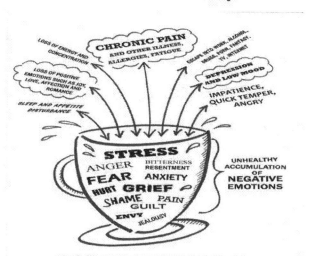

A picture paints a thousand words

Within the Chrysalis Effect approach practitioners like myself use the Wellbeing wheel (or '8 Elements of Freedom') to help us target and monitor treatment. This is a self-scored measurement tool, used to first indicate which areas need the most attention and then to monitor where you are at various points in your recovery.

8 Elements of Freedom

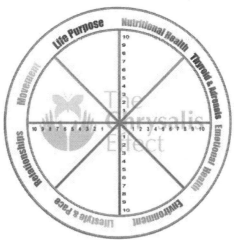

Figure 27 The Wellbeing Wheel

Tackling the lowest points in your wheel means the therapy is therefore holistic, targeted and specific to you. There is no 'one size fits all' here. There is trial and error, adjustment and patience. This is the basis of holistic therapy as opposed to conventional treatments. Finding your own answers with advice from those who have trodden a similar path and good therapists helps to keep you focused and out of your own anxiety loop. This is vital to recovery as otherwise you are bound to follow your own habitual patterns of behaviour which are likely to be anxiety driven and unhelpful.

For people who have CFS and Fibromyalgia like some of my clients, this approach allows us to begin to address the multifarious causes based on the most significant for that person. For clients like one of my Fibro clients, who had had the condition for 20 years, this was a vital missing link in the puzzle. Remarkably, nobody up to that point had every sat down with her and explained how the disease develops (via the 'domino effect' of causative factors linking one to the other) or how to begin to reverse it.

PART THREE The symptoms of stress and trauma in the mindbody

CHAPTER 8: COMMON SYMPTOMS AND CASES

In this section I will look at some of the common manifestations of trauma by looking at examples from people who I have seen in my clinic. I don't claim to be exhaustive therefore. You are referred to books in the reading list for more detailed considerations. I start with some of the most common and work through to those that are less so. I describe examples from my clinic of people who have come in with a variety of diagnoses (or sometimes no diagnosis at all) to show how the commonalities outweigh the differences and, in reality, it is not the diagnosis that is the issue but what is happening in the person's life before and concurrent with the symptoms. Invariably there is some experience(s) which has not been processed properly which is contributing to symptoms. I hope that by showing the diversity and subtlety of the symptoms you will begin to understand the nature of trauma and recognise its effects in yourself or those you care about.

Depression

Depression has become so endemic in society that it has become common; scarcely anyone has been untouched by it in some way. Anti-depressants are the number one prescribed drug in the UK with "half of women and 43% of men in England (..) now regularly taking prescription drugs" to combat it, according to the comprehensive Health Survey for England[84]. This constitutes a considerable burden on the NHS (where the cost is paid for through taxation) as well as intense suffering for those thus prescribed. We may have reached a situation where we are both "over-diagnosing and over-prescribing" according to author of that report, Dr. Clare Gerada. Although the report stresses that there are things we can do to help ourselves, including eating well and regular exercise, no-one mentions releasing trauma either directly or indirectly as a source of relief from depressive symptoms. This is a failure of understanding and of service provision therefore.

It has been my experience, and that of many of my clients, that access to mental health resources are meagre and sporadic, with many people being referred to group stress management courses as the only recourse available on the NHS (i.e. publicly funded as against privately). Whilst these are helpful they do not solve the ongoing problem of unprocessed memories as the wellspring of stress and depression. This understanding of implicit memory formation is simply not that well known, even in mental health services. Trauma as the source of the problem, despite being so prevalent, is ignored.

Much research effort has been devoted to working out the underlying cause of depression, with particular focus on changes in neurotransmitter levels. Up until very recently it used to be thought that depression was simply a lack of the neurotransmitter serotonin so the new class of anti-depressants SSRI's (Selective Serotonin Re-uptake Inhibitors) were developed. These acted primarily on the uptake mechanisms of the synapse (gap between neurons) to prevent re-uptake of the released serotonin thus prolonging the amount present in the system. They have been heavily promoted and prescribed to mixed results. Some now believe that they are less effective than first thought[85] and their use, although continuing, is considered risky amongst certain age groups (young people are particularly susceptible to a side-effect of mania[64] and suicidal thoughts).

We have come to the point where depression is now defined as an illness, a chemical problem of low serotonin, despite there being very little evidence of this fact as it is incredibly difficult to measure serotonin levels in a live human. We simply do not know "what is a normal level, much less what is an abnormally low or high level" is. In any case, the picture is a lot more complicated than depression being a lack of serotonin, as there is some involvement of endogenous opioids ('feel good chemicals' in the brain) too[86]. The body simply does not work with one hormone / one effect like drugs do. There is always a complex web of inter-related hormones, neurotransmitters and control mechanisms so that fine-tuning and responsiveness to changing environmental conditions can happen. The body is not, after all, a machine; it is far cleverer and more complex.

We have the situation where a theory has been elevated to the status of established fact in order to sell pharmaceutical solutions. And this strategy has been marvelously successful with rates of anti-depressant prescribing growing over 400% in the US since 1988[87]. Over half the patients aren't even being treated for depression but for other problems like chronic pain and insomnia. It's a seemingly unstoppable juggernaut.

The result of creating this new disease category is that we promote a one-size-fits-all solution of the 'magic pill'. It's as if people exist in an experiential vacuum where what happens to them to cause the depression is simply ignored. At no point are we encouraged to look at our life experience, belief systems and coping mechanisms. Science has gone down the road of reductionism, where everything is reduced to its smallest components in the hope that we will one day find the biochemical cause.

But we ignore at our peril the psychology of a person and the social milieu they live in. These are important considerations as we have seen and may help us devise a more holistic healthcare regime with lifestyle adjustments and self-help strategies.

It has been shown that exercise, play and perceived social support are, in many cases, more effective than SSRI's via their epigenetic effects on transcription i.e. turning certain genes on or off. So it seems that encouraging self-efficacy (enabling people to learn new techniques to encourage hopefulness and providing support for change) might be essential factors in the success of therapy, regardless of particular technique used. I cover this in more detail in the case studies where a variety of different techniques are used to help people recover. Essential in my approach is encouraging people to develop their own expertise and to practice 'new ways of being' outside of the therapy room. For instance, I suggest they get in touch with their creativity and take up dancing or singing to help reduce the stress response. To the medical establishment it may seem a bit 'new-agey' but when you understand the science behind it, i.e. bringing the right brain and left brain into better communication, you see that these things are really a vital component of therapy, particularly with highly traumatised people whose prefrontal cortex has gone 'offline'.

Getting people to look at their 'map of the world' for errors of thinking such as distortion, generalisation and catastrophising is an important component. Thinking, as we have seen, is a habitual response to certain perceptions. If we see the world according to our map, we tend to follow certain stereotyped behaviours based on those beliefs. If we believe that people are always out to get us or 'life is difficult' we tend to interpret people's behaviour towards us that way. According to some spiritual teachings we attract more of the things we focus on (Law of Attraction[88]), so if our overall impression of life is in a frame of scarcity, hardship, and victim status, that is what we will find. Henry Ford once said "whether you think you can, or you think you can't--you're right." It's all about belief.

One of the main factors in overcoming depression is tolerance of uncertainty[89]. Life will always give us challenges, but how we overcome them is often based on knowing where we can intervene and where we can best leave well alone. Human beings are hard wired to analyse; we want to understand why something happens, and with some life events (death being a very good example), we simply cannot know. People can agonise for a long time about what the 'right' thing to do or what the truth of a situation is and the brain, being a pattern-matching organ, will obsessively try to figure it out to the point of exhaustion.

My overriding aim when working with depressed people is to find out what, exactly, they believe about a situation and help them to firstly notice those thoughts, and then, ultimately to challenge them. Engaging people to believe in their ability to actively *create* their life rather than being subject to the unknowable whims and fates of the universe is what gives them resilience and strength to change. As an example, working with someone after a relationship breakup, we isolated that her overriding belief was 'this always happens to me'. When we looked at the situation however, we found that in the current breakup, the situation had been very different to past situations and, in fact, she had far more clarity and self-determination than before. By showing her also how to 'act powerful' using social scientist Amy Cuddy's 'power pose'[90], we managed to change her physiology to someone who feels grounded and connected. This enabled her to get her through a potentially difficult meeting with the ex-partner where both of them came out feeling empowered and shame was banished. It worked. She quotes "I was calm, mature, reasonable and I even managed some humour". She also reports she cannot believe how different she feels in such a short time.

Changing your outlook and way of being in the world can very effectively manage depression, but you need help to do it as it is almost impossible to analyse your own behaviour. Engaging the body is also absolutely vital and is often forgotten. Depression often goes hand in hand with physical pain and not only because being in pain is depressing! For reasons we've explored already "depression, like most persistent pain, is frequently a manifestation of an underlying emotional cause"[91]. But by seeing depression as only a 'mental health' problem though, physical solutions are often ignored. Yet many patients who consult with this problem will have many other issues; digestive difficulties, unexplained pain, insomnia, etc. This is simply ignored as an anomaly, and the patient (you) continues to suffer. We need to look at depression as a symptom of something unbalanced in all three realms of wellbeing; mind, body and soul.

Anxiety/Insomnia/ Panic Attacks

Anxiety

Anxiety is another of the common diseases of modern life – often co-diagnosed with depression although in fact they are opposite ends of the arousal spectrum. Anxiety tends to occur when you are hyper aroused (in the amber zone). As you are in fight or flight pretty much permanently it is hard to think straight as your thoughts go round and round in interminable circles (called rumination) which serve only to make you more confused and stressed. Anxiety states cannot be dealt with simply by medicating as, although, the drugs may help in the short term they do nothing to treat the underlying cause which, as you've probably guessed has emotional trauma at its core. Psychotherapy is needed, particularly that which looks at unconscious process (depth psychology). If you can't afford professional help then there are some excellent self-help strategies out there online. I highly recommend an Australian CBT-based site called Moodgym which helped me considerably.

But as with depression, we must approach it with a mindbody perspective and help to engage the resources of the recoverer and not the sufferer. This may involve finding time for mindfulness, meaningful connection with others, being outdoors in nature and other simple solutions while you explore the deeper reasons why you are being triggered. Try to examine what you were doing prior to particularly anxious times. Use journaling to highlight patterns – they might give you clues as to what could be causing your feelings to escalate.

Also note that anxiety can sometimes present itself as a distraction, when you are beginning to make the connections with stress and chronic pain. In other words you start dealing with the pain, and anxiety may then manifest more acutely. The mindbody knows it's 'number is up. It is important to acknowledge that the anxiety is just another symptom of stress and is not an indication of mental instability. You have to be kind to yourself and allow yourself to release the judgement that somehow it is further evidence that you are defective!

Insomnia

Due to the high levels of cortisol running through your body when you have anxiety (especially late at night) it makes it very hard to sleep as cortisol is the main hormone for getting you awake and buzzing (remember the circadian cycle from Chapter 5?). The downside also is that getting up in the morning is hard too as instead of being high at this point it is too low so you are sluggish and non-responsive. You enter a downward cycle as "the less sleep the more cortisol" is produced[92]. So insomnia may become a pattern, particularly if it is developed as a problem in childhood (as it was with me). Even now, a problem that is out of my control will keep me awake most of the night. I find it very hard to switch off a response that was developed in my early years.

Insomnia may be the first sign that things are not as they should be in your life. Our bodies need restorative sleep for repair and renewal of body tissues. However, worrying that you are not sleeping is counter-productive so it is best to try to keep to the cycle that helps you (late sleeping if necessary) and just accept that even lying with you eyes closed is better than nothing. You will read in other books exhortations to go to bed early and keep to a routine –which may work for some people. But for those with chronic insomnia and fatigue issues it is hard to give up the pleasure of suddenly feeling better late at night when you are finally able to do all the things you have been unable to in the day.

I would certainly agree that keeping to good 'sleep hygiene' rules (darkness, no stimulation after 9, no wi-fi, laptops, TV's and other Electromagnetic Frequency producing devices) is a good idea, particularly for those of us who are highly sensitive to such things. But, more importantly I think is what you do with the time you have and what you tell yourself about your problem sleeping. It is extremely important to stop blaming your body for 'failing you'. This message is a very common one for highly driven, stressed people who are showing the first signs of chronic stress states. Because your approach is one of being super conscientious, with your self-worth tied up with being 'productive', any failure to keep going is produces a deep sense of shame and anger. I remember feeling that way, where I would berate my body for letting me down, and then push it all the harder the next day and the next. It is no wonder I collapsed with exhaustion.

The answer to this self-perpetuating cycle of stress and blame is, interestingly, *play* and creativity. The first thing that you have dropped probably when things started to get difficult and the last thing on your mind when you are feeling exhausted at your lowest ebb. But play you must. Whether it be singing, dancing, drawing or reading a good book, you must put back into your life those right-brain activities which allow your analytical brain 'time off'. Allow yourself some pure relaxation time too, where doing nothing is a purpose in itself. Go on try it. I know its difficult when your whole life may have been about how much you can achieve. Whatever you choose to do, make it meaningful to *you*. What you do is not what's important here, it's what it means to you to do it. So if volunteering, fishing, or singing in the church choir give you a buzz then follow that. It may take some detective work as you've likely forgotten how to play. Check in with yourself what you loved to do as a child and do more of that. And if you're really stuck, just try something that you've never done before and see how it fits. I have clients who really have no idea what I mean here and they have to 'dig deep' to find out what they love. They've never even given it any thought. A very sad state of affairs.

Panic attacks

Panic attacks[1] are an extreme form of anxiety that manifests as a physical response to fear in the form of rapid beating of the heart, palpitations, sweatiness and dizziness amongst other things. The body feels like it is in preparation to run (which in fact it is as it is 'fight or flight' mode) but it can feel like you are having a heart attack or dying, which is not the case. The trouble is you may have no idea why you feel this way as the panic may have developed due to an unconscious trigger which as we've already discussed may be associated with the initial situation that created it. Hence you have no conscious recall of either the initiating event or the association with the trigger. All you know is your body feels in great danger.

I had a client recently who was about to go on holiday but was having very mixed feelings as she has lost her father recently and she was about to return to his former home in Italy. This manifested in a very physical way as odd sensations and aches in her back and down her legs. Now, you will know by now that I am very much a believer in the mindbody connection. I told her it was very likely that these odd pains were linked to her imminent departure but that she should get checked at the doctors just in case. The doctor gave her a clean bill of health so we were left to work on the symptoms from a mindbody perspective.

According to my experience and Sarno's work, it seems that the mind will create aches and pains to distract you from the more painful and serious *emotional pain* that you are trying to avoid confronting. I know if you haven't come across this idea before it may sound strange but time and time again I have proved this. Anyhow, it seemed a classic case to me as these pains had come on suddenly a few days before her intended departure. In our therapy session we started with EFT which allows you to both own the symptom but also release it. As we worked together I saw a wave of emotion appear to come from her stomach (where she had located the current pain) and wash over her face - tears soon followed. There was a tremendous amount of grief pent up in this person, which she hadn't really dealt with. Or, more correctly she has deal with it consciously but the subconscious had not and thus was still stuck with the loss.

At the heart of these symptoms was emotional conflict. Leaving to go away was both pleasurable (it was a holiday after all) and painful as it was

---

1 During a panic attack the person "often fails to discriminate between body sensations of arousal or movement and emotional feeling, which can lead to the escalation of both". Their interoceptive sensitivity is heightened by trauma which means they both feel body sensations (including pain) more acutely and they interpret them more negatively. In short, you panic about panicking.

the place she had last seen her father AND in order to go she had to leave her elderly cat who was also very dear to her and possibly wouldn't survive. This is a classic case of internal conflict; you both want to do something and you don't want to. The guilt and conflicted feelings come out with back-ache or sciatica or whatever. How can you tell if what you have is a true pathology (i.e. structural problem) or a mind-body issue? Chase the pain. What I mean by this is use the EFT protocol (detailed and described in detail on my website to apply the tapping protocol and see if the pain *moves*; it usually changes in some fundamental way pretty quickly.

For my client, I had instructed her to do this the night before she came to see me as it would give me a strong clue as to whether to treat the pain with physical or mindbody therapy. She reported that it went from her legs to her stomach. So, I had a pretty good idea we were dealing with a mindbody problem[1]. In the therapy we did together the pain moved again from tightness in the stomach to a constriction in the throat (interesting as this often reflects something unspoken). As we continued this developed into a full blown panic attack so I asked her to move to the table and we worked on calming the autonomic nervous system with belly breathing (which helps to break the shallow breathing /oxygen deprivation cycle triggering panic in the brain) and then I helped her speak her pain and then we shook her limbs to release the pent up emotion[2]. I find it helps people to experience their emotion through their body which is where it resides. There is much theory around how the mind and subconscious process interact. I have included some more information on my website.

Suffice to say I was successful in this treatment and my client left - shaken obviously but no longer having the trauma in her body. Her pain disappeared immediately and she sent me a text from holiday saying how much she is enjoying herself. (Though it's worth noting for accuracy that she did experience another panic attack at a subsequent time - one session is not going to undo 40/50 years of trauma!).

Chronic Pain, Fibromyalgia and Chronic Fatigue

This group of disorders all have common symptoms; pain and fatigue usually alongside depressive symptoms of insomnia, anxiety, digestive issues, sensitivity to light and noise, and other symptoms which you may now be able to understand given the effect of trauma on the body (vagal

---

1 Dr Daniel Clauw calls this 'Centralized Neuropathic Pain'. He maintains that the fact it is multi-focal pain (i.e. that moves around) is characteristic of centralised 'brainpain' and not tissue injury.

2 this approach has been detailed in Peter Levine's work – see his books Waking the Tiger and the more recent Healing Trauma

innervation remember?). Hyper-sensitivity is your norm and the more you have it the worse your symptoms are likely to be.

Chronic Pain

I deal with a lot of clients who suffer from Chronic (persistent) pain of one form or another, who may not have had a proper diagnosis – although by definition chronic pain is considered to be the relevant diagnosis once pain has been present for more than 3 months. Chronic pain differs from Fibromyalgia and Chronic Fatigue Syndrome only in the fact that fatigue is not a major part of the symptom picture. However, in my experience they are on the same spectrum, often arriving after a significant period of stress and not responding to physical treatments.

I have recently been working with an older lady who suffered terrible back and leg pain (diagnosed as 'sciatica'[1]) which she was convinced had come on after a doctor had given her anti-depressants. She believes that the pills were directly responsible for the anxiety and pain that she felt as the pain came on suddenly afterwards. She had no previous experience of pain. However, after taking a thorough case history it appeared that her life had been one of quite significant trauma. She had been married to a chronically depressed man, who was very controlling and emotionally abusive. She had had a forcible abortion due to being misdiagnosed with cervical cancer and had grown up with a mother who was not in the least maternal or supportive. The symptoms that this lady experienced had come on after her husband had died and this seemed to me to be very significant – often conflict may show even in potentially positive experiences – she was free to be who she was at last! But of course guilt and regret then came into the picture. Not to mention anger. It doesn't matter to her that she nursed her husband for years, she still finds herself facing intolerable emotions of relief that he has died and terrible guilt for feeling that way.

My first priority with a client like this is to stabilise the anxiety cycle from continuing to trigger more pain. I do this with EFT and psychoeducation explaining the mindbody theory of the causation of pain by unresolved emotion. Although my client had not heard of this theory before she began to understand the links with her personality and life history. Once we have begun to take the focus away from a structural cause and looked at the traumatic events in her life, we can target those with EMDR treatment. I do also look at physical therapy of course, mobilising

---

1 For many years it has been understood that sciatica is where the sciatic nerve which runs down the back of the leg and is impinged by the vertebral discs or by 'piriformis syndrome' where it goes under or through the piriformis muscle in the buttock and get's entrapped when the muscle is tight. The reality may be more complex with emotional factors of amplification in the picture too.

the tissue with massage, relaxing the body with Reiki and encouraging dietary changes like juicing and cutting down gluten and dairy (ideally we eliminate these altogether). Finally I recommended daily infra-red saunas[1] which have very good results with chronic pain, reducing lactic acid formation and generally encouraging detoxification.

Often just acknowledging that you have emotions that are not being expressed is enough to reduce the pain for some people. With this client her life history was such that she had never had the chance to express them and would actively repress anything emotional as 'silly'. Her language was full of self-deprecation 'I'm stupid and weak', 'it's my fault I'm this way', etc. Or paradoxically they can look to demonise one person or situation that 'caused' the problem. In both these examples we need to take the emotional punch away from these negative thoughts to move people on to focus on recovery. I liken it to a pressure cooker that has the heat turned up but the lid on. We need to release some steam (acknowledging we have some unacceptable emotions – guilt, relief, anger, etc) and then tackle the subconscious drivers providing the 'heat' (I'm unworthy, unlovable, pathetic, etc).

In the example with this client, she had just got to the point where life was promising for her after her husband died. After years of being abused and restricted she was now free to explore who she was. Her considerable conflicting emotions of relief, and then painful guilt were difficult to tolerate; instead of acknowledging those unacceptable feelings she channeled them into anger at some perceived external threat (the uninformed doctor who 'did' this to her) by prescribing 'dangerous pills'. This is how the psyche works; I call these endless ruminations 'toxic thoughts'. My client particularly identified with this concept – this made sense to her as she recognised the cycle of negative thinking and worry that had brought her body 'to its knees'. Sometimes just explaining what is going on can intervene in the anxiety cycle enough to break it and pain to be released. However, more often the client will have to learn all the ways in which their habitual thinking and established beliefs have contributed to making them ill. This requires practice as these patterns are well engrained in the neural networks so will need rewiring.

In this case it has been significant that all of the bad interactions my client has had with the medical establishment have been with male clinicians. The problem is that throughout her whole life she had been subject to the opinions and domination of her husband, and other men,

1 Infra-red wavelengths have been shown to be extremely beneficial in reducing incidence and severity of chronic pain as they gently heat the tissues and release toxins.

even well-meaning clinicians, simply triggered that memory. The fact that they rarely had time for her or gave her experience credence was also a factor (she was dismissed as a 'neurotic woman' by many). She finally found a female pain specialist who patiently explained what could be causing her pain, giving her time and a physical explanation which she found very helpful. At our last appointment she was visibly beginning to take back control and is, I believe, on the road to recovery.

I had one impromptu 'client' at a Wellbeing Day I exhibited at recently - she was another therapist who was interested in trying a taster session of EFT as she'd heard of it but had never tried it. Ironically, she couldn't think what we could work on as she'd 'sorted everything' previously with other therapies. I asked her "is there anything troubling you today?" to which she replied "well only this nagging back pain" so we decided to work on that. I decided to use a protocol called Faster EFT™ (see later) with a few extra touches of my own, as it's such a quick and incisive tool. In fact within minutes I had this poor lady in tears as she reconciled the fact of not loving or forgiving herself for stuff that happened to her in childhood. I had not expected to go so deep so quickly but then I am not in control of what comes up. All I can do is allow the self-directed process to begin – the brain knows what it needs and is very intelligent about taking you to it. We allow the process in and out of the recall of traumatic memory (so-called 'pendulation') to be always under the client's control. I hold the space and engender trust that their brain/mind will allow them to move through it. A feeling of safety is paramount and must be created beforehand and throughout.

As this lady wiped away the tears and I gently held her hand, we repeated the mantra 'I am safe'. This may sounds airy-fairy nonsense to some of you A-types out there (and I am one so I know), but please believe me people who have been traumatised often do not feel safe at all – anywhere. They have constructed very careful personas to avoid facing that reality –they are often highly competent and hard working but at their deepest level they feel alone and helpless. It is for the reason that most therapists working in this area have had trauma themselves that makes it so important to do this work well, without getting attached to the outcome or psychologically involved. We don't want the client's trauma to re-trigger our own (and thus likely make them feel unsafe – so-called 'transference and 'counter-transference respectively). Connection and grounding are two sides of the same coin.

I watched her face all the way throughout - the facial muscles and expressions are intimately connected with our emotions - via the vagal nerve - and are very instructive. Her face suddenly looked very scared and childlike. As we worked through what had come up and gradually defused the emotional charge, the adult began to creep back in. At the end of what had been perhaps 20 minutes she asked me what I saw and I told her I saw the face go childlike and then adult. She said it was very odd because that day she had grabbed a crystal (crystals are believed by some to have powerful healing energies) to take with her; the one she had grabbed that day was for 'the inner child' apparently.

As we drew to a close and I asked her how she felt and she said "my back pain is gone" and looked astonished. This is no longer a surprise to me as it used to be. I now know that emotional 'stuckness' can be expressed in bodily pain and it seems clear from the work I've done that the pain will often shift, or move or change its character in response to clearance of these old emotional memories. She walked away feeling and looking quite different. I don't know if she'll venture to come back and see me for a longer session - I can't control that but I know I did good work with her and I felt that my purpose for going that day had been realised. Sometimes you only sow the seed. Chronic Pain is unlikely to be completely transformed with one session as the pathways are so ingrained. But you can certainly make a considerable difference.

Fibromyalgia and Chronic Fatigue

The first time I encountered a client with Fibromyalgia was when a lady came to me for a massage and, although she had sought out the treatment, we both found it difficult as being touched was painful for her – excruciating in fact. It was hard to work on someone who would wince the minute I touched her and then grit her teeth through most of it saying she knew it would feel better afterwards! The muscles particularly affected are the postural muscles of the back, neck and pelvis i.e. shoulder girdle and buttocks[1]. This seems to be a common place of holding tension, as those muscles are constantly active even in rest and they are the muscles of defensive clenching when under attack. This is highly relevant to trauma of course.

I had taken a client history and she reported that doctors had first diagnosed her with 'fibrositis' over 20 years ago and it was still with her. During this time she had had the condition renamed twice! I was astounded. Here was a client who was in evident pain (you can't fake that look on the face) and on multiple medications but was evidently no better, in fact probably getting worse. Although she had seen many, many

1 Not for nothing is finding someone difficult called a 'pain in the arse'. The metaphors of bodily states are often very revealing.

therapists and consultants, done a lot of research herself online and by reading books, etc she was no nearer recovery.

This experience sent me into a tailspin. I was not used to making people feel worse (even initially). Most people enjoy massage as being profoundly relaxing not painful; in the case of fibro the muscles are full of lactic acid from poor energy metabolism so pressing on them simply releases it. But at the time I had no idea of this. I determined I was going to find out more and, as luck would have it, I found myself at a workshop at a professional therapy fair a few months later where someone was talking about chronic fatigue and fibromyalgia. I learnt that the syndrome had physical, mental and emotional correlates. People who get it tend to be A-types: hard working, driven and people-pleasing – always putting others before themselves generally. They usually have some form of trauma in their past[1] and the trigger is normally a secondary trauma like accident, infection, surgery, bereavement, etc in their present life. There will be nutritional deficiencies and gut issues but the primary driver, it seems, is the emotional memory of past trauma (often bullying or abuse) which has not been assimilated properly. This is still not commonly accepted by the mainstream.

In fact if you read some of the online information and the highly regarded books by senior consultants as I did when researching this condition, you find that hardly anything is known at all and recovery is 'impossible'[2]. The 'disease' is somehow defined by its symptoms (pain in 7/10 common areas – known as 'trigger points') and there is lots of information about how to manage it but very little description of how it occurs and why. I came away mystified as must anyone with such a diagnosis. However, I can now confidently tell you both CFS and Fibro involved disturbances to the HPA axis, cortisol levels and an 'over-activation of the amber state of fight and flight' which if not tackled leads to the red alert of the freeze response. Unfortunately having the illness itself keeps the stress cycle going and adds to the stress load, particularly if it is combined with hopelessness of ever finding a cure. It is no wonder people struggle for years…

There are certain extra considerations when dealing with people with long-standing syndromes such as these. Deeply embedded feelings of shame at being so ill and unable to function, exacerbates what is already likely a shame-burdened childhood. Coupled with this the fact that

1 Women who have been physically abused in childhood have twice the odds of developing CFS and 65% higher odds of developing Fibromyalgia. They also seem to then have bullying at school / work

2 According to the NHS http://www.nhs.uk/Conditions/Chronic-fatigue-syndrome/Pages/Treatment.aspx there is 'no cure'.

mainstream medicine tells you it is incurable and at best will have to be managed for life. Given this dire prognosis many sufferers turn to support groups for companionship and solace. But such is the complex mindset of people for whom their sense of self is so intricately tied up with achievement and success, they often begin to champion the fight against the disease itself. They do this to counter the generally held and erroneous assumption that it is not a *real* disease and in order to fight for better treatment. But it can become more of an identification as a 'sufferer' of the disease itself. Anyone who suggests it can be healed then becomes vilified in a mistaken attempt to gain back control. I myself have suffered this response when trying to help people in such circumstances. I now keep well away from such support groups, as I believe that their focus is counterproductive. In my view they are negative and part of the problem[1].

Luckily there *are* approaches which aim to help people recover, by taking responsibility for their health and beginning the work needed to recover. Most people *do* want to get better, but they use their left brain (analytical, logical, problem solving) to try to make sense of the condition, where in fact it may be more helpful to re-connect with their creative, intuitive, body-orientated right brain selves. I always suggest going back to doing something that you loved as child, having regular bodywork, improving your nutrition with extra B-vitamins, Co-enzymeQ10, omega-3 fatty acids and magnesium *and* getting in touch with your emotions via journaling. Then I suggest one of the many self-help programmes like the Chrysalis Effect or the Natural Health clinic. These all share a multi-modal approach i.e. body, mind and spirit are tackled. So, it just doesn't fit the medical model of increasing specialism and reductionism which is why the two approaches seem worlds apart.

CFS has been covered in detail in the previous section as it encompasses many of the features of Chronic Pain syndromes. Indeed, along with Fibromyalgia it could be called the 'poster child' of mindbody pain syndromes. It is a multi-faceted disease which requires the same treatment as Fibromyalgia as they are but alternate manifestations of the same thing.

Dissociation/depersonalisation

Whether one has suffered the trauma of abuse or the more cumulative low key trauma of rejection or poor parental attachment, dissociation is often the result. Dissociation (a feeling of being outside your body) is a

---

1 There are of course some wonderful exceptions out there where disease is seen as complex and involving psychological factors and whose approach is one of recovery. But they are the exception.

necessary response to a situation that the person finds completely intolerable. It may be temporary e.g. the person feels as if they are floating above their body whilst the event is happening, or time slows down and gives you an altered perspective. This normally resolves itself when the danger has passed. However, if the dissociation is very severe it may become a permanent state which interferes with the person being able to inhabit their body and 'depersonalisation' (a state of being disconnected from a sense of self) may result.

There are many different terms used for dissociative disorders which range from minor, transient states to the more severe Dissociative Identity Disorder or DID (which used to be called multiple personality disorder). They all share certain characteristics of trauma-related symptoms which cause alterations in the way the brain co-ordinates its activities so that there is a discontinuity in the sense of self. They run along a spectrum with mild dissociation at one end (very common), through PTSD and finally with DID at the other with a prevalence of being about 1-3% of the population[93]. DID is distinguished by the lack of integration of parts of the personality so that each part is unaware of the other. It is NOT about multiple people sharing one body which is why it has been renamed. It is a failure of various brain circuits responsible for a subjective sense of unity. DID is often a result of early attachment failure with disorganised attachment being the biggest predictor. But other diagnoses exist with lesser symptoms such as common trauma and other unclassifiable dissociative disorders which may explain some of the physical symptoms I see in clinic.

Whatever, the diagnosis (and there are many in the latest psychiatrists' diagnostic manual, the DSM-V), I look at it as a *survival technique* rather than an illness. It enabled the person to provide psychological distance from otherwise unendurable trauma. In therapy I am keen to help clients focus on the clever way that the mind has devised of keeping them safe. Getting engaged with this aspect of survival switches off the traumatic 'back brain' and switches on the 'front brain' (cortex). We take the high road rather than the low road[1]. This acts as an antidote to the powerlessness of being locked into inhabiting a diagnosis (i.e. I *am* dissociated, I *have* dissociative identity disorder).

This may seem disingenuous but actually, it is a necessary precursor to getting the person involved enough with their own symptoms to care. Getting curious about how the mindbody has (mal)functioned is absolutely

---

1 Researcher Joseph Le Doux was the first to coin these terms which distinguish the slower cortical structures (the high road) from the faster survival brain (brainstem and limbic system – the low road).

essential as it brings the cortex online again and allows the person to begin to see how their mindbody has created this as a response to a particular set of circumstances. People with these disorders, like those with chronic fatigue often, believe erroneously, that it was one event that caused their illness; whereas I see it as the 'straw that broke the camel's back' i.e. it was the final event in a series of sensitising events that finally overwhelmed the mindbody. 'With unresolved trauma the brain hasn't registered that the trauma is over' and people are hypersensitive to the onset of each new threat.

People with this condition may well have always struggled with being social in larger groups and found that they retreated into their own quiet world to survive. Of course social anxiety is common, even among those of us who consider ourselves mentally well it is quite a stressful thing - it's just that most of us are clever at hiding it! For trauma sufferers it is completely intolerable. They cannot even work up the courage to walk into a room where there are large numbers of people. They find it difficult to distinguish the sound of someone talking from the general noise around them (this is due to a malfunction of the thalamus which filters incoming signals and the insula which controls selective attention, and having complex relationships becomes fraught with difficulty.

The sad thing is that with this degree of dissociation, the sufferer does not feel real in their body, and their interactions with others are superficial. One client told me the only reason she could come and see me is that I look like a 'cardboard cut-out' to her so she doesn't believe I'm real either. I felt inclined to show her I have three dimensions and am as real as the chair she is sitting on but as nothing is real to her that's a pointless exercise. So you can see it is the brain's perception of reality is altered and makes functioning extremely difficult. People with these conditions often have poor digestion, with severe constipation and/or diarrhoea depending where on the arousal scale they are (amber = diarrhoea). Because nutrition (and in particular good nutrient absorption) is needed for recovery this is an added problem.

It is vitally important to feed back to these clients that the problem is in their *perception*, not the reality. The reality is that their body still notices everything that happens to them, and responds to it. But they are simply not aware, the disconnection is between the sensation (and the feelings that these engender - usually fear) and the interpretation by the brain (meaning - e.g. I am in danger). I always stress that the disconnection they feel is ultimately a safety valve for the feelings that have simply become intolerable. Particularly when the feelings are ones of rejection and humiliation (shame) from those who are meant to love you; those feelings are simply unacceptable and are disconnected from the mindbody completely.

So, when you understand the dissociation as a symptom of your trauma, and the degree and timing of it, the labels no longer matter so much. They are just defenses your mindbody has erected. They can be dismantled and re-programmed but very, very gently. This degree of spiritual disconnection from your own body cannot be solved easily and may take years.

The usual approaches to trauma, like EFT and EMDR are difficult to apply as the person is asked to concentrate on their feelings as a precursor to both techniques which is almost impossible for them. So, although I do use these, I have to allow the person to gain confidence in trusting their own body not to betray them first by:

- Psychoeducation – showing how the mindbody communicates and how trauma works to change the balance of the body.

- Bodywork – breathing, massage, progressive relaxation, walking, meditation, etc

- Pendulation – being able to feel and to think at the same time by grounding with tapping (not the full EFT protocol), and other psychosensory approaches bringing you back to your body gradually.

One of the techniques I have found especially useful in the beginning is applied kinesiology - it has a huge following in chiropractic circles where it is used as a sort of communication system with your subconscious. I find that very interesting but, more appropriate for dissociation disorders is learning to use it psychologically. Check out the videos from Bruce Lipton and Rob Williams called 'The Biology and Psychology of Perception'[94]. I hope you find they inspire you as they did me. Both men are respected in their individual fields; Bruce in particular is a cell biologist who has garnered many awards for his insights. His book 'The Biology of Belief' is required reading for anyone interested in the mindbody link although strangely it is still classified as 'alternative' despite his scientific credentials.

Finally, it's worth noting the more naturopathic interpretation of rejection causing dissociation is that you have a deficiency of spleen energy - apparently there is a link between the spleen and rejection[95]. I am constantly amazed by how many conventionally trained doctors and other clinicians are finding truth and answers in the more esoteric fields of 'alternative' health. In any case I am aware that when solutions that work are not accepted by the mainstream it is usually because the model is wrong[1].

When people tell me that such and such has no proven method of working I remind them that neither have SSRI's or anaesthetics. We still don't know how they work really.

PTSD, Flashbacks, recovered memory

My first experience of encountering trauma in the therapy room began when a new client came for a massage, and, as she was lying face down on the massage couch and I lightly touched the back of her neck, suddenly began to sob uncontrollably and choke. I was aghast - I had never encountered a flashback before. Somehow at the back of my mind, I knew it was nothing that I had done and tried to keep calm. Despite having no experience of this (they don't teach you to watch out for this in massage school!), I managed to use my innate wisdom and hold her gently by the shoulders and reassure her with the words "you are safe, you are here with me" and she eventually calmed down and was able to tell me what had happened.

Lying face down triggered a memory of an event that happened to her when she was very young – perhaps 2 or 3. She was sexually abused by a relative and held down on her front. It was the associated body (procedural) memory of being in that position that was triggered by lying on the couch and my simple (and benign) touch. Remember, the explicit (narrative) memory is not possible early in life before the brain is fully developed (hippocampus is not online) so that events like this are coded wordlessly in sensory fragments. At this age the survival brain is in charge, the cortex is effectively 'offline' until about the age of 7- 9, and so implicit or wordless memory is more likely to survive unprocessed by cognitive understanding. If the event is very extreme or persistent the mind will resort to dissociation (splitting off) of the event entirely. Dissociation, then, is a failure of memory processing.

The dissociation that occurs when a very traumatic incident happens is a protective mechanism, to enable the child to survive such an extreme event. We often say a 'part' of their personality breaks off, many victims report floating above themselves viewing the event from above. This is because the situation is intolerable to the psyche if it stays integrated so separation is needed for survival. It is one of the reasons why memory of abuse is often forgotten until later in life when it is safe to recall. This is what happened to

---

1 In fact this is a classic Type II error of research where we miss the detection of a real phenomenon because we have false beliefs, or inadequate methods to evaluate them so we ignore those facts that do not correlate with our model. Jaak Panksepp outlines this in detail in his book The Archaeology of Mind' P11. Meridians, energetic medicine and such may well become accepted practice in the new paradigm of mindbody medicine when/ if we are able to measure them.

my client.

This disturbing incident which shocked us both was the beginning of working together on a deeper level. But first I had to learn more about trauma and how to treat it. My instinct luckily had been spot on – reassuring the person to keep in the here and now when reliving trauma and instigating a sense of safety are all vital components. We have to re-work the trauma so that we don't panic and can make a realistic assessment of what is going on – we are 'making the implicit (amygdala) explicit (hippocampus)'

Recovered memory has a chequered history, with controversy in the 1990's fuelled by the increase in compensation claims by people claiming to have been abused. There was much disagreement about whether memories can, indeed, be effectively repressed or forgotten this way. Although opinion was divided amongst the mental health community (psychiatrists, psychologists, etc) then, it has now become clear that early memories *can* be repressed as a safety device by the brain to avoid overwhelming events. We even have a mechanism for this; with stress causing the hippocampus to go offline through the effect of cortisol[1]. In fact this is a normal part of traumatic memory formation as we have seen in the science section. Freud viewed it as too damaging to the logical part of the brain which he called the ego. Modern theorists such as John Sarno see it as more of a protection mechanism, of which pain and physical symptoms may be the distraction from uncovering emotional feelings.

Skin problems: eczema, psoriasis, scleroderma

One of the things I began to notice with a lot of people who came to see me for stress-related problems was the preponderance of skin issues, particularly psoriasis or eczema. Conventionally, these are regarded as different diseases, but both primarily of inflammatory origin. For several of my clients, the continuous scratching caused more itching and bleeding which was a source of considerable shame which just exacerbated the problem. One of my first massage clients had extensive eczema on his body which he could handle until it occasionally spread to his face. Then he avoided contact with people until it subsided.

I began to wonder though, as I studied the history of these clients (mostly women), if poor parental attachment might be a common link. Most seemed to lack safety and security in their parental upbringing; often the mother who is primary particularly in early life, but often compounded

---

1 Cortisol is highly toxic to the hippocampus and it becomes much smaller as a result by up to 20%.

by a complicated bond with the other parent who may be absent or the relationship compromised in some way. It was not that the parents were necessarily abusive – in fact often they were 'regular' parents – but as we have already seen trauma is not necessarily the result of severe experiences but the cumulative experience of more minor ones. And being emotionally unavailable or erratic as a parent means your child cannot rely on safety. As one of the leaders in the field of trauma, Bessel van der Kolk has said 'the most severe dysregulation occurred in people who lacked a consistent caregiver'[96].

As we have seen, trauma has direct physiological effects on the body and the stress cycle may create an inflammatory cascade of neuropeptides throughout the body[97], which may be expressed in the skin. If it is very severe it may develop into the more serious auto-immune condition of **scleroderma,** a potentially serious condition which involves over-production of collagen in the skin and elsewhere. There is often a co-presentation with Raynaud's syndrome (see later section) and digestive disorders, particularly Gastro-oesophageal reflux disease (GERD). Like both of these and the other conditions mentioned in this section, it affects predominantly women, usually between the ages of 30 and 50, and has no known cause (conventionally). Unfortunately, it can become systemic affecting the internal organs and is therefore considered a serious disease which can be fatal. People who are diagnosed therefore, are often considerably stressed by the diagnosis as they are told there is nothing that can be done. I would highly recommend getting together with a positive community of fellow recoverers as I recommended with Fibromyalgia and not giving in to fear. All auto-immune conditions come and go with stress and adding to the burden with doom-laden prognoses is not very helpful for the person suffering. Diet is also key here as the skin is the largest organ in the body and is often the first to be affected when detoxification processes are compromised[1].

I had one client who had the compulsion to pick and scratch her skin, particularly on the eczema which she has had for a long time (see skin section for more information on why this is common). In some ways this is no different from cutting, though obviously a milder form. Whatever is under the surface of her mind is making her anxious, and the act of physically hurting helps to assuage that feeling with a surge of endorphins. The person who has just self-harmed is then rewarded by feeling better and

---

1 You may read in the press that detoxification of the body is not necessary as the liver does it all for us. This is true in an ideal situation. However, when the liver is compromised as it often is with modern diets and stressful lifestyles, the skin often has to take over and is often the first sign..

the act of conditioning begins where that action is encouraged by biochemical changes in the brain (largely Dopamine, DA, release).

We cannot approach this problem consciously. She is under no illusions that the damage this does is anything other than destructive – in fact it makes her angry that she does it so she can be, like many others, trapped in a cycle of self-loathing, which makes her more anxious, which increases the urge to do it. A rational, highly successful person in all other areas of her life, she is mystified by her actions and wonders if hypnotherapy will help.

My approach to this is first to discover what the underlying cause is and it transpires that attachment trauma (a mother who failed to bond well with her) has set her up for sensitivity to stress which she early on had to self-soothe. Self-harm can be one of the ways that children learn to do this in the absence of soothing by the parent (see the section on attachment for more details of this). We find that the scratching is worst early in the morning and late at night when not 'distracted' by work or competing demand. This is not unusual. In fact, by this time I am beginning to see the itching itself as a distraction produced by the body to hide the underlying emotional pain that is present, but cannot be felt (it is suppressed as being unacceptable – being 'weak' is not something this client sees herself as and she has conflated the emotions of childhood with weakness. Sadly, although her childhood ended a long time ago, and she is no longer dependent on a emotionally erratic mother, her belief systems were encoded then and so she responds as if they were current.

During hypnotherapy, I decide to use a version of parts therapy which views the mind as composed of competing parts which are failing to communicate well (in fact we now know that this is neurologically closer to the truth than we thought – via the corpus callosum which joins right to left brain). During the session we as to speak to the part that is controlling the picking behaviour and we ask it to describe what it is trying to do for her (we always start from the understanding that the mind always has a positive motive, even for what seems like destructive behaviour).

We are both surprised when the 'part' explains that it is trying to contain the 'heat' in her body which looks like little hot coals with arms and legs which come towards her. Scratching gives her something to make the coals run away. She feels she is walking on 'hot coals' always (a great metaphor for being with a bipolar mother) and impressed when it comes up with the solution of painting some blue cooling paint both on the coals and on the part of her body that is itching the most (her feet, not surprisingly). This painting that we do is itself a metaphor, which is how the subconscious often likes to communicate. Afterwards she seems astonished that we could have a communication with a part of herself that she wasn't aware was there, and how childlike it was. It is an extraordinary experience to do this, when your life is lived in the conscious mind only, it's like waking up to the 'child within'.

After one session, she reports that the itching has lessened and the urge to scratch is gone. There is more work to do, I'm not going to pretend that was it and it disappeared forever, though that sometimes happens. This was a person who had gone through a recent severe trauma, and we followed up with some EMDR to work on that. The feet, I can now report are a lot healthier and she herself feels a lot calmer.

Addictions

In many ways addictions are a re-playing of early survival mechanisms. After all a child mostly needs love and attention; and when we cannot find what we need, "we feed ourselves what we can find"[92]. When you understand the mechanism of addiction as being a powerful neurochemical hit of dopamine as a 'reward' when the person obtains their 'fix' (whether that be drugs, drink or the more nebulous addictions of picking, nail-biting, etc) in the face of anxiety, it is no wonder that addictions are hard to kick. We are hard-wired to seek the thing that reduces our stress, even if it kills us. I have no experience of working in the traditional addictions field but I find many people that come to me with chronic conditions and dysfunctional behaviours often share a similar outlook of obsessive behaviours. They have been repeatedly told to abstain as the solution, when in fact they need to clear the trauma that causes the behaviour.

One of the best ways to overcome the addiction is to look at the underlying message; what is it doing for you? We can explore this in hypnotherapy where we may replay the scenario that leads up to the addictive behaviour and practice doing something differently, or we may explore in more detail the notion of 'parts'. In many ways this understanding mirrors the dissociative phenomenon we explored earlier although in this case we are seeing parts as not separate identities but as different aspects of the same personality. If we understand that we all have parts of us with differing needs, it gives us a way of exploring that part and what its use is to us. We all know that certain behaviours have different motives. For instance with the example of someone who is nail biting for instance, this distracts attention from being looked at, it gives us something to 'do' when we are anxious. Being overweight may give us the protection of not being desirable, drinking gives us more confidence.

However in parts therapy we take it as a given that there may be more than one motivation behind an action – we often talk colloquially of this when we say something like 'a part of me wanted to and the other part resented it'. However we can work much more directly with these deep psychological drivers when we undergo hypnosis and allow the subconscious parts to be more readily available to enquiry. When we give the parts a colour, name, quality it makes them more tangible and enables us to talk directly to that part. This may sound odd but once again, we are dealing with the subconscious parts of your mind rather than the logical conscious. The subconscious is communicated with in metaphor – rather like in dreams. If we engage directly with the part and ask it what its purpose is and whether it can think of another way of achieving the same end, surprisingly, this is usually spontaneously available in the mind of the person.

Unless you have undergone this yourself I appreciate this may sound very strange indeed. But the power of hypnotherapy is that the metaphorical constructs of the human mind become the tools with which we work rather than the logical, language-based elements. I have had much success with this method of deconstructing the various conflicting reasons behind a particular action and finding alternate ways of dealing with the issue. Once you get all parts to agree, you can often find the urge to engage in your addiction is lost, or at least very much reduced. Finally then you can deal with the reason you initially found the behaviour comforting, whether it be intolerable feelings of anxiety, abuse or simply boredom. The aim is to understand, and re-target the behaviour by changing the underlying feelings.

Anger (Defensive Rage)

Anger is a normal emotion when it is temporary and resolved, helping us to overcome difficulty and provides drive and motivation. But it can become traumatically encoded and disabling. For some it is too unacceptable an emotion and will be repressed – this could be deemed to be one of the differences between men and women (although I have seen women with a lot of anger and men totally unable to connect with it at all). I had a client who demonstrated how this can be expressed as a result of trauma. He came to me because he was suffering depression but his was of expressing this was unusual. He had begun to notice he had extreme reactions when driving, and an extraordinary number of road rage incidents. It had begun to scare his partner and his daughter as, although he hadn't actually hit anyone yet, he had come close on a couple of occasions and upset an elderly couple who dared to pull in front of him without signalling properly. Most of us have this experience from time to time, and I guess, if we're honest we've also done the same to others in periods of inattention. Usually this is greeted with a bit of swearing and we move on. But my client seemed unable to do this, he exploded when anyone crossed him (as he perceived). He seemed completely unable to control these outbursts and it would plague him for days.

He also seemed to have problems in work relationships too, and had been involved in a serious accusation of bullying at work. His gentler, vulnerable side was clear to me from our discussion but it was not one he found it easy to engage with when triggered by stress. In treatment we discovered some deep issues with attachment to his mother, never having felt secure or understood. His mother continues to trigger him even in adulthood by sending inappropriate texts or ringing him to demand attention. He had had to move away from his home country in order to escape her overbearing personality.

Early on in life he had made a pact with himself never to allow anyone to get the better of him, as his experience of never being good enough for her made him feel terribly inadequate. This may have saved him as a child but it was an inappropriate behaviour now which was making life hell for those who loved him. The use of anger to re-enact confrontational scenarios is well known to therapists who work with trauma. The modus operandi of people whose failure to bond to their parent(s) is a form of dissociation. To not be present emotionally makes them seemingly invulnerable to hurt. But once set in motion that way of being becomes habitual and they find it hard to connect with others emotionally. This makes for poor trust in relationships although they may be fully successful in other areas of their lives, often choosing professions that are dominated by logical, left-brain thinking. The difference with men and women here is where they then direct their inappropriate emotions. Men tend to direct outwards and women inwards, although as I have said before these are generalisations and there are plenty of examples of people who cross the gender stereotypes. Much depends on your personality structure.

My client learned where his anger came from and, with targeted EMDR on some core 'touchstone memories', was able to begin to connect with his sadness and loneliness as a child. By showing himself compassion he was able to forgive his mother and see her inadequacies as a result of her poor parenting[1]. He went on to become a physical therapist himself, finding a way to use his experience to benefit others enabled him to heal his wounds in a daily, practical way.

---

1 Forgiveness is about letting go of the holding pattern yourself not condoning the actions of others.

IBS

IBS is a common complaint consisting of periods of constipation and/or diarrhoea. It is twice as common in women as men and prevalence is estimated as between 14 and 24%[98]. This may be due to the interaction with the more delicate hormonal balance of women, particularly the sex hormones, which seem to make the situation worse particularly during the egg-releasing (luteal) second half of a woman's cycle. However the peripheral nerve contribution of the ANS are rarely considered.

The colon is innervated by the vagus nerve and is highly influenced by stress factors mediated by the HPA axis and the adrenal stress cycle. One client I had would suffer terribly when at work and then her symptoms would melt away when she was on holiday. We knew stress was a big factor but it was difficult for me at that time to distinguish between the dietary changes of her vacation with the stress-induced changes. I didn't know polyvagal theory at that time and had to rely on current diagnostic practice which relies on questionnaires aimed at categorising the 'type' of primary symptom in the expression of the disease i.e. is it primarily diarrheal or constipatory? The treatments offered are supposed to be linked to which is the dominant symptom.

However, my experience of using these symptom questionnaires is that they are a smokescreen for really saying 'we don't know what causes this' but making it sound scientific and reproducible. In fact, the way that IBS is dealt with in mainstream medicine is similar to many of these other chronic multi-factorial diseases I have described i.e. very poor with multiple medications for symptoms and little relief as the true cause is unaddressed.

Once you know that the amygdala links very closely with the vagus nerve and that subconscious stressors as well as conscious stressors play their part in activation of the alternate 'fight and flight' (diarrhoea) and 'freeze' (constipation) response, it all makes a lot more sense. Treatment within this frame of understanding will be aimed at releasing the subconscious drivers of trauma-related memory.

Meunières Disease /Vertigo/ Earache/ Tinnitus

Meunieres Disease is an interesting condition which was first described around 1860 and has been variously attributed to imbalance of fluid in the inner ear and calcium phosphate stones forming there. It is another one of those diseases, like fibromyalgia and IBS, for which the diagnosis is descriptive rather than based on an understanding of causation. It primarily affects women. Vertigo (sudden dizziness, loss of balance) is something we normally experience if we are faced with steep drop when we have a fear of heights[1]. But it may come on suddenly without this stimulus, become chronic and disabling. It is often seen alongside CFS, migraines and IBS often accompanied by ringing in the ears (tinnitus) and occasional hearing loss. This should immediately ring alarm bells with what we know already about vagal innervation. You will remember that the ventral vagus nerve (part of the parasympathetic social engagement system) innervates the ear as well as other parts of the face, jaw and neck (via cranial nerve V and the auricular nerve).

Earache is another expression of this triggering. It is commonly seen in children due to infection (**otitis media**) but with adults, once other issues like infection, and so on have been ruled out, it is deemed to be 'psychogenic otalgia'[99] with unknown cause (i.e another psychosomatic or mindbody phenomenon). I suggest that these conditions could be linked to undischarged traumatic memory being triggered subconsciously and habitually via vagal nerve stimulation. This would explain both the symptom variability and the co-occurrence.

It is most certainly a stress-related condition as we see that substances such as caffeine and high salt intake (which cause changes in blood pressure) and simulate sympathetic nervous activity all make it worse. What makes it better are steroids (= synthetic cortisol, the parasympathetic hormone) and, not surprisingly, stimulating the relaxation response with yoga, meditation and the like. What I would like to see added to that list is emotional (implicit) memory resolution which I have demonstrated has beneficial effects.

Tinnitus may also be considered a symptom of unresolved conditioned and unconditioned stimuli which sensitise the system to 'initiate a vicious circle of "overexcitation of the auditory system"[100] with many similarities with central neuropathic (i.e. centrally driven chronic) pain. In that sense all these seemingly unexplained symptoms may belong to a family of sensory mis-firings from unresolved procedural memory.

Raynaud's disease

Another syndrome which baffles medical science is Raynaud's - over-sensitivity of the peripheral blood vessels (arterioles) of the fingers and sometime toes. It is often called 'white finger' as this is the main sign as the blood supply is cut off from the tips of the fingers. It is particularly seen in cold weather (cold is a stressor which activates the stress response), but with people who have it very badly, it can happen even in the freezer

---

1 Fear of a 'falling horizon' is one of the naturally encoded fears in the human species.

section of the supermarket! I get it in the index finger of my right hand and nowhere else. It began in my thirties alongside depression and digestive issues. When it was first labelled by a friend of mine as a 'disease' I was aghast. I had always thought of it as simply something strange about that finger, much like having one that is bent or big ear lobes (both of which I also have). I had no idea it was a symptom of an over-responsive nervous system that affects the small blood vessels response to cold temperatures.

The arterioles are controlled by nerves of the sympathetic system and are a normal part of the fight and flight response to restrict blood flow where it is least needed[1]. The problem is it becomes over-reactive and will be engaged even when not needed. Again it tends to correlate with stress-related and auto-immune disease (particularly scleroderma) which have a lot of the same precursors as many of the chronic fatigue-related diseases (leaky gut, excess toxins and inflammation). It certainly responds to hypnotherapy approaches of warming the hands by biofeedback (you imagine your hands getting warmer whilst engaging your subconscious). Again I cannot definitively link this to trauma but my experience and those of my clients would suggest that dealing with the trauma in order to clear emotional issues may have unexpected side benefits of reducing these and other physical symptoms.

Accidents, drama

You may be very surprised to find this listed in the common manifestations of trauma but I have found this so often it can no longer be deemed co-incidental. People with a history of trauma seem to have more accidents than others. One of my clients had no less than three serious motor vehicle accidents (MVA's) in the space of 5 years. Another had a serious accident the day before she was due to come and see me! Each one, of course, produces further trauma. You could argue that when people are distracted and/or ill they are more likely to have accidents, but it seems that the causes are a deeper malaise. The Law of Attraction (which I cover in more detail in the next chapter) would deem that you were simply attracting more of what you focus on, and helplessness and lack of control would seem to find its epiphany in an MVA. But I believe it may be that people unconsciously attract scenarios close to the originating one as a process of re-enactment. This is understood within psychology to be the compulsion to re-enact the trauma[101], whether in relationships, habitual behaviours or

---

1 Dr Bruce Rind and other nutritional therapists believe that adrenal insufficiency coupled with heavy metal toxicity also plays a part being stored in the finger tips where they will cause least damage.

addictions.

Whatever the cause, it seems clear that excess stress and anxiety tends to increase the likelihood of unforeseen events and drama in one's life. I myself had a history of such events; before I got ill with CFS I had my first vehicle repossessed for a debt that wasn't mine, with the loss of £20,000 and six month's income while I struggled to take the criminal to court[1], three MVA's – two where I hit pedestrians (who crossed in front of me without looking) and one near-miss on the motorway. All of which occurred in only 8 years of driving. Since resolving many of my subconscious traumas I have not had one event in nearly 15 years (not to tempt fate..). There is much that can be done to examine the patterns of drama in your life – the so-called 'drama triangle[2]'. But you may need to work with a competent therapist to really clear the deeper-seated ones. Once you do so, the energy of that uncompleted stress response is no longer trapped in you creating havoc in your life.

---

1 This case would be funny if it hadn't really happened. I bought a car off a guy privately, subject to the usual checks by the RAC, but at that time didn't include leasehold vehicles which this turned out to be. The company whose car it really was eventually tracked me down 18 months later, waited until I went on holiday and then repossessed it leaving me with a black bin bag of my contents to come home to. I never recovered that loss as the real criminal who sold me the car had a heart attack on the first day of court and died. The strain of that process then precipitated the loss of my relationship.
2 First developed by Stephen Karpman, MD in the 1960s as a psychological tool to analyse the roles of Persecutor, Victim and Rescuer, it has become part of family therapy and transactional anaylsis.

PART FOUR Treatment Approaches

CHAPTER 9: MINDBODY SOLUTIONS

One day medicine will be unified - it will stop seeing things as compartmentalised into physical or mental realms and realise we are mind *and* body and one affects the other in profound ways. We will stop looking for the magic bullet of chemical medicine and look to supporting the body's innate healing powers instead – possibly by looking at the biophysics (quantum mechanics) more than the biochemistry. We are at the crossroads of a new medicine with insights into the nature of DNA, which we now know emits biophotons at a rate invisible to the naked eye but detectable to very sensitive machines via bioluminescence. This radiation may actually be the basis for information transfer more than the chemical nature of the repeating base pairs in the sequence. After all, we still don't know what causes DNA to be read in one particular way which creates a human, as opposed to a mouse[1].

This bioluminescence may correspond to the 'auras' visible to some people (whether through accident of birth or perhaps practice). Energy transfer may explain the meridian lines of chi known to Eastern medicine. My experience with Reiki early in my therapy career was extraordinarily challenging to my Western, scientific training and yet I can no longer deny that it is real. I can 'feel' (sense/detect) areas of the body that are troubled (by doing a body scan where the hands are held over the body). I feel it as a pressure wave and it seems very accurate. When I reveal my impressions from scanning to the client I am working on, they usually admit knowledge of something wrong in that area and are very surprised that I can tell without touching. I find the more I hone this sensory awareness the clearer it gets. I can't explain how this works using conventional scientific understanding, but as I've said over and over in this book, we may simply be missing the point. When our model can't explain what we witness in everyday practice, instead of re-configuring the model, we say it can't be happening and deride any further evidence of such[102]. We have so tied ourselves to the mast of so-called 'evidence-based medicine' (EBM) founded on lab-based clinical trials, that we have ignored a huge part of that evidence base – clinical experience *in our clinics*. This bastardised version of EBM has been hijacked to a very narrow interpretation which benefits Big Pharma and excludes so many useful therapies and non-patentable products e.g. herbs.

---

1 Rupert Sheldrake, author of A New Science of Life suggests it may be due to 'morphic resonance' or the collective memory of a species being shared by a quantum effect of information transfer.

I hope that the medicine of the future will use some of the advances in modern medicine but do so in a more intelligent, integrated way incorporating knowledge from psychology and spirituality. These aren't flaky ideas. They are being proven time and time again in myriad ways in labs and clinics across the world. Even something as simple as essential oils can be extremely powerful anti-cancer agents, for example, and have been proven in study after study[1], but you will seldom hear about them in the mainstream press because they don't fit the model of the magic bullet promoted by the pharmaceutical industry and their paid up research colleagues. Don't be persuaded to give up control of your health until you've explored this 'alternative' vision. It has much to teach us.

We have been given some wonderful new tools by people working in a more holistic, integrated way. Some are therapists and clinicians who have discovered new techniques. Others are Western adaptations from Eastern approaches. Whatever you choose and however you decide to go forward, just *do* something. Take responsibility for your own wellbeing and be proactive. Understand that we are entering a new paradigm of health where being the passive recipient of 'treatment' is no longer an option. When it comes to these complex conditions we need a much more integrated multidisciplinary approach.

My overview of what is available to us that follows is not meant to be comprehensive. I have deliberately kept to tools that I use or have experienced myself. I know there are many other options out there and I would encourage you to explore them. However, the main point is, you no longer need to suffer. There is a solution and it's up to you to find it for yourself. You may wish to get help and, of course, there are real benefits to working with a good practitioner who can help guide you to wellness. But it is a collaborative approach, one in which you will be asked to be an active participant rather than passive. You will find that your mindbody knows far better than you do what it needs.

Holding the space; creating safety and empowerment

An essential precursor to working with anyone who is willing to come for mindbody therapy is that they begin to *take responsibility* for where they are in their lives. Please note I am not saying take the blame. Remember responsibility is the 'ability to choose your response'; it is wholly different. When people begin to see how their whole lives have been a precursor to this event (the illness or whatever), they are able to finally begin to forgive themselves, forgive others who have done damage to them, and eventually

---

1 Frankincense oil, known since biblical times, is one of the most powerful chronic stress and anxiety relieving agents, reducing pain and inflammation, boosting immunity, and even fighting cancer.

take responsibility for their own lives and heal[1].

So this does not mean apportioning blame to oneself or anyone else. It is about gaining perspective that your genetic tendencies, personality, life experiences and environmental triggers combine to create the situation you are in. Your beliefs, forged as they have been in the crucible of experience, are largely a construct which help you to defend your idea of yourself and your personality. Many theorists including Freud and others, such as the metaphysician Marianne Williamson, have called this the 'ego'. More recently Eckhart Tolle[103]. author of the highly influential 'The Power of Now', has referred to it as the 'pain body'. It is so much a part of you that you have probably never examined it before, never seen it as separate from you at all. You have become your thoughts and beliefs, both psychologically and physically. Your subconscious communicates and interacts with the body throughout your life. But as you have never been taught how to listen to this innate wisdom and focused instead on using intellect and the constructed shields of your particular personality type (over-working, judgemental, self-critical for instance) to protect you; you have never accessed this deeper self-knowledge.

Not only might your innate psychology have worked against you but you have been culturally trained to accept a disenfranchised view of life. You have unwittingly gone along with the conventional view of illness which told you to think of illness as being a chemical imbalance requiring a chemical solution only to be provided by 'expert' clinicians with access to the right drug or treatment. This view has entrenched your powerlessness, locking you into a constant search for the miracle solution, which usually ends in defeat. Philosopher of science Karl Popper called this constant promise for the magic bullet 'promissory materialism'[104]. It's like having faith in something that is based on belief rather than reality — like credit is to banking[2] - it has no substance in itself. With modern medicine we are constantly hearing that the miracle treatment is 'just around the corner' but it seldom appears. It is no wonder most people are made more anxious by their condition, feeling that there is nothing they can do.

By changing the way you frame health and illness, I help you see it as a *process* rather than a single event, and your disease as something that started as a spiritual crisis long before it showed up in your body. When you feel defeated / overwhelmed by life you will tend to need quick answers, and something to blame for the situation you find yourself in. My approach

---

1 Healing is not the same as curing. You may not overcome your illness totally but you will use it to become more whole; your condition becomes your teacher rather than your punishment.

2 And we've seen what happens to that with the recent 'credit crunch' creating global havoc.

encourages you to recognise your situation as a result of *everything* that has gone before, and embrace acceptance and willingness to change. Here, your relation to your environment, specifically your relationship with your therapist is *key*. By creating a safe space for you to reflect on where you are currently, you can look at your strengths not just your weaknesses. You can see how your behaviours and beliefs helped you survive up to this point and appreciate how powerful you actually are in this moment, creating yourself anew with every thought you think. Finally you can take control of your life in this awareness and now choose to do things differently[1]. When clients get this, there is an 'ah-ha moment' of revelation as a huge weight is lifted off their shoulders. They are powerless no more.

So, the actual approach is not so important as the belief the client has in the treatment[2], the qualities of the therapist and how empathetically they respond to the client so that the client feels both heard and valued. This 'holding the space' is vital so only work with someone who you connect with in this way. It makes the therapy so much more powerful.

Psychotherapeutic approaches; Psychoanalysis, Hypnotherapy, Mindfulness

Psychoanalysis

Within psychotherapy there are many different approaches, of which few seem to totally agree with each other. Sigmund Freud was the first person to really study the psyche, from which he developed a model of the mind and treatment of neurosis which he called **psychoanalysis**. His tenets which he developed in the 1890s still hold remarkably true[3]:

It is past experience in which there may have been one or more traumas which is the root cause of a person's current problems.

- The personality is developed early in life – specifically early childhood.

- Human behaviour and thus experience is driven by unconscious drives.

- Attempts to reveal these drives are met with resistance which may be in the form of repression of certain memories.

---

1 It may seem simplistic but often awareness precedes change. Most people are simply unconscious in their lives, and bringing them into awareness is often enough for them to make profound changes.

2 The 'placebo' effect whereby a sham treatment, offered in a believable way, can still be effective.

3 Freud also developed some now discredited ideas such as sexual longings of the child for the parent. It seems he formed these theories based on the rejection of his early ideas that many adult neuroses were the result of child sexual abuse. Viennese society at the time could not countenance this idea as it was too shocking so he was forced to change his view. We now know he was right and child abuse was rife amongst the upper classes as it was the lower.

- Conflicts between conscious and unconscious can cause mental neurosis, anxiety and depression
- The mind uses various defensive strategies[1] to keep the primitive, guilt-inducing emotions out of consciousness using repression. This takes much energy to maintain and does not contribute to good psychological adjustment. Therapy is devoted to encouraging the conscious expression of this unconscious material via abreaction[2].

However, the kind of therapy that this encouraged could be extremely long-winded with sometimes a life-long commitment! Luckily, that is no longer considered necessary. Cognitive Behavioural Therapy (CBT), which came to prominence in the 1990s, remains the dominant school currently as it has the best evidence base for success. However, whether this is because it is the best method or is simply the best researched remains a moot point. I think it is very successful in some areas where habitual negative thinking is the problem. My training was largely in this method and its framework is one that I favour because the main focus is to enable people to build self-efficacy rather than to continue re-living past trauma. It differs from psycho-analysis in that it isn't interested in going over past experience but is more concerned with your current interpretation of that experience.

By looking at your *thinking* (or cognitions) around your situation, it aims to reframe them in a more accurate (and hopefully positive) way. I still use this CBT model as a basic framework for working within. However, as you might imagine from the argument I have presented here, there is a limit to how much we can change with thinking when some of the causative events are wordless sensations in implicit (wordless) memory. Hence I do believe, along with a number of other clinicians / researchers that you can't change the feelings by talking about them. You have to evoke the feelings (light up the neural pathways) before you have any hope of changing them (reconsolidating the memories). So, in trauma therapy particularly, we need a different approach.

Hypnotherapy

Hypnotherapy has a problematic public image. Firstly it is associated with TV shows where hypnosis is portrayed as some sort of magic mind-bending trick. Clinical hypnotherapy is a world away from the showmanship

---

1 Including chronic pain.

2 Here I differ from Freud- it is not necessary to 'abreact' (expose, express through re-living) an event. It is necessary to feel the emotion though but this can be done without describing it.

of those sensationalist TV hypnotists. It suffers from many misconceptions based on public ignorance. One of the main ones is that it is something that is 'done to you' by an all-powerful therapist. That couldn't be further from the truth. Most hypnosis is self-hypnosis and part of the process is to practise some of the techniques at home until you become proficient. In common with most successful therapies, it involves a joint commitment to work together with the therapist and homework is part of developing your sense of self-efficacy. It is a combination of hypnosis with psychotherapy.

Secondly it has struggled to be accepted within the profession of psychotherapy in much the same way that homeopathy has within medicine. It remains to this day classed as 'alternative/ complementary' medicine even though it has huge efficacy in areas such as behavioural change and pain management that far surpass many more conventional approaches[105].

This is an accident of history. Had Freud continued in his exploration of hypnosis we might have a very different psychiatry profession today. Initially he was very excited by the possibilities it offered and, along with Pierre Janet and others, found it to be a very effective treatment for all manner of 'neuroses'. He later abandoned it in favour of other techniques like free association and automatic writing, and, such is his legacy, that we have a situation today where it is not considered mainstream therapy, but something a bit risky. This is a shame but understandable given the misinformation and lack of support for the technique within the medical profession. I do understand the reticence of people who are ignorant of what it involves as I was one of those people myself before I learned the techniques.

Hypnotherapy is not, as you might imagine, scary or weird. It is actually really practical as it involves accessing the subconscious part of the mind more easily as we disengage the conscious process a little. This can be by creating a relaxed state or by changing the object of focus away from the incessant thinking to the body. We can begin this process by asking someone to focus on relaxing one muscle at a time as a scan through the body. This progressive muscle relaxation allows the client to gain control over what has been previously unconscious – and to realise their state of constant tension!

Acceptance as we have seen is key in all forms of recovery. In this state of deep relaxation we can present ideas to the subconscious that which would normally be difficult or frightening. An exposure therapy technique called systematic desensitisation uses the fact that it is psychologically impossible to be relaxed and tense at the same time. As we present the idea of something the client finds difficult (e.g. feeling fear), we start with just describing it, and then we go in more detail until we get the person to engage with the feelings in their body but all the while encouraging them to feel totally relaxed. As we allow them to process the fearful thought without feeling the fear in their body they gain mastery over their feelings and we break the anxiety cycle which is often a bodily response to 'fear of the fear'. However, there may be limitations in this approach with severely traumatised people and trauma specialist Bessel van der Kolk warns 'desensitisation is not the same as healing'[106].

There is another benefit within trauma therapy "as it can be very helpful to those whose nervous systems are in a state of hyperarousal to concentrate on a tiny part of themselves that might not feel as difficult – it might be their big toe, but with that you have the possibility of beginning a process towards a calmer state, even from such a seemingly small place, it is a beginning. It is not that you negate the part of you that feels difficult, you hold both together in your awareness. It might be that 95 percent of your system feels unbearable but there is 5% percent that does not, you accept them both and the process begins."[107]

Hypnotherapy accesses subconscious process in a way that talk therapy finds more difficult and time consuming. It is like a shortcut to the deeper part of your psyche – in this way we talk of it being a 'depth psychology' tool. What I love about it is it uses metaphor and guided visualisation to 'tune in' to the deep-seated beliefs and therefore behaviours of a person without needing many hours going over the events of their lives. This is very important for traumatised people who are likely to be re-traumatised by recounting difficult events. Milton Erickson was one of the most famous hypnotherapists who used stories and metaphor to subtly challenge the belief systems and internal mindmap of the client. Others have used more physical methods to temporarily disengage the mental defenses such as distraction and confusion. Whatever method is used, they all have one thing in common. They are working subconsciously with the psyche which, as we now know, is the biggest part of our brain and the most involved with traumatic memory. As such I find that it speeds up the process of recovery hugely and is a mainstay of my approach.

One of the most exciting benefits of hypnotherapy is in changing the brain, which is highly relevant to chronic pain syndromes. There is a very direct effect on the brain's interpretation of pain and dysfunction, which as we have seen, is a very big part of many of these chronic pain syndromes. Since most of them are not a problem in the periphery of the body where the person perceives the pain, but in the central nervous system (brain and spinal cord) where pain is interpreted, hypnotherapy is a very powerful tool for changing those pain amplification pathways. Indeed we can use the brain itself to change the brain which is mind boggling when you think about it. Using a subconscious process we can desensitise those nerve pathways in the brain which are adding to the pain perception. If we metaphorically liken pain perception to a needle on a dial, we use our imagination to reduce the setting on the dial and, remarkably, the pain levels can drop substantially. This has been proven in trials with cancer patients for instance[108]. But I believe we can do far more with this technique and it has become the 'umbrella' within which I use all the other techniques.

Journaling

This may sound like a strange heading in a section on psychotherapeutic processes but it really is a most important one that you can do for yourself. Journaling involves writing down some of the feelings that have been bubbling around subconsciously and as such helps to reduce the stress response quite significantly. It is pretty much a constant of the various treatments I offer. It may not be constant, in fact it can be more beneficial at the beginning as people come to realise how much they have been bottling up. It may provoke a very strong reaction when it is suggested. This is precisely the point; that 'what you resist persists'. By writing things down they are no longer bubbling around in your brain causing mayhem. It may seem ridiculous at first to begin writing your thoughts and feelings but as symptoms reduce you begin to realise the power of this simple act.

Writing as opposed to talking or thinking seems to be a physical experience as much as a mental one. Seeing the words on the page can be very cathartic. Sometimes I may encourage drawing too as this engages right-brain activity. Different people respond in different ways depending on how they are wired; whether verbal, auditory or kinaesthetic (touch oriented). I hear many and various reasons why it can't possibly be of benefit to them, but once people overcome their resistance and have a go they find that it can be very powerful. It also acts as a good measure of progress which they can revisit from time to time to see how far they have come.

Mindfulness

Recently there has been much talk about mindfulness, firstly as a type of meditation and latterly as an adjunct to therapy itself. Mindfulness, which came from Buddhist philosophy, aims to effectively retrain the mind by being present in the moment rather than judging the past or fearing the future. It thus aims to prevent you **catastrophising** a worst case scenario from past experience, by merely noticing your emotions/sensations without judgement. If done successfully it enables you to retrain your mind so that you become the observer of your experience rather than *becoming* becoming the experience itself; i.e. your situation is not *you* but separate from you. Thus trauma therapists encourage a distance between the doing and the being. Life experience then becomes full of wonder rather than a burden.

For example if something causes you to be fearful you can notice that fear and get curious about it. It is important to notice without judgement. Judgement makes every emotion so much worse have you noticed? "I'm feeling afraid – I shouldn't be feeling like this! I'm so weak – grow up!" (Also notice the tone of the voice – it may sound like a parent or someone else in your past). Get curious and start to see what's happening as information rather than disaster. When you view your experience through this lens you are less likely to get caught up in it and therefore more able to gain perspective. An emotional reaction (to a person / situation) may be just a symptom of an emotion from the past – the job then is to find the root rather than judge the person who has triggered you. In fact, I often tell my clients that the people who trigger them most are their greatest teachers. That's a hard one to hear.

Mindfulness does help people come out of the anxiety cycle which contributes so much to these chronic disease states that I have described. By gaining distance from their situation they bring more of a logical, calm perspective to bear on it. You are never in a good frame of mind to make a reasoned judgement when you are feeling emotional. Emotions and stress generally hijack the thinking cortex as we have seen. If you can't find perspective immediately take time out of the situation if you can – and *breathe*. Give yourself a count to ten for instance before hitting back with a pithy attack, wait 24 hours before sending that angry email. Marianne Williamson, metaphysician and spiritual author, always says wait three days as she believes this is time to consult with one's higher self (and we all have one apparently!). She means, of course, the part of us that isn't the hurt child inside. I always know when I'm coming from that place as I find it hard to get my words out or make my point, I stammer and flail about emotionally. I can feel butterflies in my stomach and heart. I feel exposed, raw. When I feel like that I simply know that I'm not going to be able to deal with it well, particularly as the other person is likely to be feeling the same and isn't going to be rational either. The point is to firstly recognise it and then secondly wait before attacking back. If necessary ask for time out, or be honest and say you need to think about what they've said.

I won't tell you lies about how easy it is to do this – in truth it's very hard indeed. But it's a *practice* not a quick fix. You have to repeat this over and over before it gets hard-wired in – and then remember that the more threatened you are the more primitive the system that takes over so it becomes even more difficult in very emotional charged situations, say with a partner or parent. So, practise with the ones that aren't so important: the shop assistant who is nasty or unhelpful, the customer care department who show no signs of understanding your problem, or the old lady who harangues you on the street randomly[1] . Avoid the temptation to hit back as you end up driving each other into further shame. No wonder we struggle in personal relationships![2].

There is one practice that I encourage as a route to wholehearted living and that is to keep a gratitude diary or specific time of day to express gratitude. The research on this is very positive. The vulnerability and shame researcher Brené Brown has discovered that people who adopt this practice in their day to day lives avoid the fate of most of us, which is to find that our joy is tinged with foreboding. In other words whenever a good thing happens, we always look for what is lurking round the corner to dim it. I realise I've had that trait the whole of my life. I thought it was normal. If things are going well, I am already playing in my head what could go wrong. Instead, now I make a point of mentally listing 3 things that I am grateful for in that day. It doesn't stop me finding things difficult too but it keeps me from creating more of a story around it which further traumatises me. As a highly sensitive person (HSP)[109], I need to spend more time taking care of my emotions and my environment than most people. Most people with childhood trauma are like this but we live in a world where constant stimulation is the norm. Mindfulness and journaling are ways in which we can take time out and recover our balance.

The basis of much trauma therapy is the opposite to these 'top-down' (i.e. mind-led, cognitive) processes and uses the body as its starting point – i.e. 'bottom-up' processing. Hypnotherapy could be said to straddle both.

---

1 This happened to me one day outside the bank where a random stranger accused me of cycling on the pavement but she wouldn't stop shouting at me. When I got to work I was so upset – it seemed so unwarranted. I was embarrassed, shamed and humiliated in front of all the other shoppers. What's worse was that I actually felt guilty that I had done what she said. On reflection later I decided that I must have triggered her from another event and that rather than back down she had to keep going to avoid her own shame. And that is how it works in an argument. Something similar once happened to me. Who ARE these people?!

2 For an excellent rendering of the shame issue please see the excellent books and videos by Brene (accent on e) Brown: see the book list at the end or check on youtube. Does DB give any advice on how to deal with haranguers?

But there are some more recently developed forms of therapy that have revolutionised trauma therapy. They work from the body up to the deeper subconscious parts of the brain, with, eventually, an involvement of the thinking cortex. It is these to which we turn next.

Somatic Therapy; Bodywork, Yoga, Tai chi, breathwork

Somatic therapy exists in many forms, some with trademarked names like Sensorimotor Therapy™ (ST) and Somatic Experiencing™. What they share in common is they approach the body to attain psychological trauma release. They use the fact that our primary attachments are memorised in the body as feeling states and thus to transform these we must use the body to connect and release them. As Pat Ogden who developed ST has said, *"In our bodies, in this moment, there live the seed impulses of the change and spiritual growth we seek, and to awaken them we must bring our awareness into the body, into the here and now". We are seeking a twofold change: that of allowing the body to complete the energetic resolution of an action, and in that resolution, to release the energy contained in that traumatic response, allowing that experience to be perceived as one in the past. Without resolution in the body we cannot get release, as that is where it is stored (via its link to subconscious procedural /implicit memory). I see a lot of people working on spiritual awareness who ignore their bodies completely. The true health-seeker cannot do this.*

Bodywork; Fascial Release

Bodywork encompasses a broad range of treatments from massage through to physiotherapy and **fascial release**. This uses touch as the primary means of engaging with the body. It seems to be not just t the act of touch, but the quality of the touch that is important. Specifically it is the rhythmic, repetitive strokes that seem to have the most impact. "The field of restorative neurology has for many years emphasized the positive impact of repetitive motor activity in cognitive recovery from stroke. This principle suggests that therapeutic massage, yoga, balancing exercises, and music and movement, (...) that provide patterned, repetitive neural input to the (...) would likely diminish anxiety, impulsivity, and other trauma-related symptoms"[110]. Why might this be? Well it seems that the skin receives touch neurologically as information and thus the intentionality of the touch might be important.

Recent work by Leon Chaitow[111] and others has shown that the body is not a passive mass of organs and tissues but an interconnected 'biotensegrity' system of fascia. Fascia is the web of connective tissue that links all the organs and tissues like a stocking. There has recently been an explosion of interest in fascia with research showing that we need a much wider definition[1]. It used to be thought that this was merely a support stocking holding everything in but recent discoveries have shown us that it is a fluid information system called Anatomy Trains[112], much akin to the Chinese meridian lines of acupuncture, that are acutely sensitive to the outside world. For instance, the discoveries of researchers at the Arizona School of Medicine (an ostpeopathic school) show us that a change in the mechanical forces applied to tissue through bodywork practices such as fascial release or massage alter the gene expression of a cell via cell signalling behaviour[113]. We have covered epigenetic expression already in this book, it is the latest in a long line of extraordinary recent discoveries which alter our view of the human body forever. Here it seems is a direct way of altering cell signalling via *mechanotransduction* (the generation of an electrical response from mechanical touch) towards an anti-inflammatory response which has huge implications for the reduction of disease risk[114] in the human population. Most disease, we are discovering, is inflammatory, even cancer, heart disease and Alzheimer's.

Yoga

Yoga you will have likely come across, although some miss out on the spiritual aspect of its teachings; in our 'quick-fix society' we are seldom still enough to tune inwards. Yoga has a long tradition in the East, however as it is commonly taught in the Western model, it is more seen as a gentle exercise workout, and not perhaps the real mindbody connection that it should be. Yoga works on several levels simultaneously; physically it tones and stretches the body, mentally it encourages stillness and body awareness, spiritually it connects you to something greater than yourself. Its part in therapy has perhaps not been so well explored although it is now integral to many of the programmes run by trauma centres in the US and, more recently, in the UK[2]. It is not a religion, or treatment in itself; more a way of

---

1 'Fascia' now has a wider definition: all the collagenous-based soft-tissues in the body, including the cells that create and maintain that network of extra-cellular matrix (ECM), all the tissues traditionally designated as 'fascia' in classical anatomy plus tendons, ligaments, bursae, and all the fascia in and around the muscles. It has been said (by whom?) that we don't have 650 separate muscles but 1 muscle in 650 different fascial pockets. I suspect this is true and would explain how pain can transfer

2 Khiron House, London and Oxford has been set up by former trauma sufferer and entrepreneur Benjamin Fry. It is offering therapies modelled on the work of the Trauma Centre in Arizona where he had to resort to travelling to after he

life that is in harmony with nature and each other.

Tai Chi

Tai chi has a long history also but is more focused on movement to connect you to your body. The flow of chi (or universal energy) is understood to be encouraged by set movement patterns. For me these were hard to learn and reminded me too much of dance moves that I had to memorise in school. Ridiculous I know but that's my experience – some people find it profoundly calming and, of course, it has been very important to the Chinese who developed it. It is seen as a practice for life, and you often see older people doing it in parks and public spaces in China.

Chi Gung

Chi Gung is a variant of Tai Chi which similarly uses movements but these are adapted to the specific energies you want to enhance or calm. Medical Chi Gung uses similar methods to Traditional Chinese Medicine (TCM) to diagnose and then encourage the person to follow certain movement patterns based on that diagnosis.

For people who find physical exercise difficult (such as the ill and elderly), these sorts of movement therapies are powerful. Next we turn to the methods that I particularly favour as they straddle the divide of mind and body and thus help people to connect; psychosensory techniques.

Breathwork

If you have not come across this before, it may be a surprise to you that there are approaches to healing which focus purely on the way we breathe. We have already learnt that the breath is one of the ways the ANS balances itself on a moment by moment basis; with every breath in you activate the SNS and with every breath out the PNS is activated. How we regulate these two arms of the ANS controls how well our body functions, including not just our heart rate and oxygenation but the acidity of our blood and stress hormone levels. If our breathing is short and ragged, or predominantly from the upper chest rather than the diaphragm as is often the case with stress, then our nervous and hormone systems cannot be in balance. We are over-oxygenating our system with the resultant blood acidity, and long-term health problems that brings.

There are various schools of breathwork, from simple yoga exercise ,mind-bending Holotrophic Breathwork[1], to the very powerful physical

---

suffered...? when he suffered a breakdown and could find no solution in the UK.

healing modality of Buteyko breathing which claims to be able to reverse chronic disease[1]. In my clinic I use simple breathing techniques as an adjunct therapy rather than a pure modality, as I find the psychosensory approach more powerful for trauma-related issues. I assess clients' breathing patterns and we practice a more healthy pattern. Returning a person to the method of breathing they used when young (from the belly rather the upper chest) can help to calm the system and send the right 'message' to the body. But it needs practicing as most people have lost the habit.

Psychosensory Therapy; EFT, EMDR, Applied Kinesiology (Psych-KTM), Matrix Reimprinting and Havening[115]

I have grouped these techniques together under the category of psychosensory therapies as they each involve some element of sensory stimulation. Some people term them Energy Psychology (EP) as they believe the underlying change is at the energetic level of the human (considered to be energy lines or meridians in Eastern understanding or auric fields in some Western). The mainstream Western medical community does not accept this understanding at all and for a long while EP was considered 'woo woo' medicine until the research showing its efficacy began to come in. There is no doubt that EP has become more traditionally accepted in the last few years[116]. Already the American Psychological Association, APA, has begun to accept EP as a valid intervention in cases of PTSD and other issues like anxiety, compulsions and pain[117].

A recent review by Brendan Murphy has shown us that good evidence is beginning to mount of the benefits and could have a remarkable effect on reducing health care costs[118]. I won't get into a full political argument here, but perhaps you can understand that there is considerable pressure to discredit these methods as 'quackery'[2] from the scientific establishment, as the drug companies consider the loss they stand to make if people were offered these techniques as a first line treatment instead of pharmaceuticals. Just a brief glance at comments on alternative health postings on youtube

---

1 Stanislav Grof, a researcher and developer of a system for inner exploration using the breath, has developed this system. See http://www.holotropic.com/index.shtml

1 Ukrainian doctor Konstantin Buteyko http://www.buteyko.co.uk/ developed his protocol in the 1950s to help treat asthma. However, the techniques appears to help many other chronic issues.

2 Interestingly the origin of the word 'quack' when applied to medicine is where the dental societies criticised dentists who were using dental amalgam as a filling in the teeth. They considered it dangerous and a ridiculous treatment when it was first introduced! How times have changed – now the dentists' professional organisations are generally in denial about the dangers and quacks are the people who oppose its use (or anything outside the mainstream). Like us!!

will show you that there is a vast army of internet 'trolls' who make it their business to post offensive and discrediting information on anything that is not considered mainstream, regardless of its research-base. The problem is there is little money available to fund research on anything other than pharmaceuticals so compared to the vast budgets of the drug research industry, there is less high quality research. However, the research evidence is mounting as some organisations and more open-minded clinicians begin to fund small-scale trials. I would ask you to keep an open mind (which after all is the true focus of the scientific method) and do not discount anything just because it is not yet mainstream.

There is scope for 'alternative medicine' to do more research to promote its methods. As researcher and therapist Daniel Siegal has noted "sensory-focused work enables clinicians of all persuasions to understand practical approaches to psychological growth". Cognitive Behavioural Therapy or CBT, although the dominant psychotherapy offered currently, is not effective in all cases and, due to publication bias, is often over-promoted[1]. This idea that cognitive functioning is the dominant means by which we function, termed 'top-down processing' (LeDoux, 1996), is based on the idea "that the upper level of processing (cognitive) can and often does override, steer, or interrupt the lower levels (...) of emotional and sensorimotor processing. Much adult activity is based upon top-down processing *except when traumatised*"[34] (my italics). Trauma upsets this universally accepted phenomenon as it reverses the process so that the upper levels are inhibited and thus become dysfunctional. CBT therapy therefore has difficulty in engaging a traumatised person.

I was trained in CBT-based hypnotherapy (CBH) so I know it can be very helpful when combined with working with the subconscious process. However, there are some limits in how effective it can be. For a highly traumatised or dissociated person thinking about yourself is almost impossible as you have no concept of inhabiting your body in any case. Thinking about the problem is of little benefit if you feel outside your body, and therefore experiencing your life second-hand. For traumatised people, as we have seen, unresolved implicit memories set them in a state of perpetual high alert. The cortex cannot function under these conditions so logic and analysis are absent. Talking about it can't touch it.

Psychosensory therapy however uses the body to talk to the mind (via the more ancient reptilian and limbic brain). This is called 'bottom-up processing' and entails some form of stimulation to the body which helps

---

1 Publication bias refers to the idea that positive reviews of a dominant theory tend to get published whilst negative reviews will not be. Hence the dogma is established and promoted.

to activate the mindbody connection (connecting the thinking and more primitive brain structures). There are two main techniques that I use: EFT and EMDR. You may find many more.

In the case of EFT (Emotional Freedom Technique) the client is asked to feel the emotion in the body whilst tapping on the face and torso. This seems to encourage certain primitive brain linkages to be made – right/left hemispheres, deep and front brain, etc). In EMDR (Eye Movement Desensitisation and Reprocessing) the emotion is discharged using eye movements from left to right and in Havening it is via touch or stroking. All have the effect of stimulating the brain in ways which we don't quite understand, although we think that probably they deactivate the limbic system which allows memory processing to be properly completed with a context stamp that marks the event as 'over'. This seems to switch on the cortex so that traumatic memory becomes logically processed as in the past and no longer threatening thus deactivating the stress response. Both EFT and EMDR share common features of approach in the therapy room but for the moment let's focus on EFT

EFT

Initially in an EFT session, I get the client to identify a problem, limitation or false belief that they'd like to work on. We rate the feeling that they get when they think about the problem via a SUD score - **Subjective Units of Distress**, measured at the beginning and then after clearance. Usually I get them to rate the score 1- 10, where 10 is the worst it could be and 0 is they can't feel it at all. Of course this is self-rated (hence 'subjective') but since we are only comparing it before and after treatment it acts as a reliable measure of the person's discomfort. We aim to reduce the score to 0 but often it sticks around 2 or 3 which usually means there are other aspects to be cleared. Working through the issue often means exploring all the facets of that problem. For instance if it is over-eating which relates to feeling fearful about getting attention then we may need to look at the fear of standing out, or being successful or whatever else is caught up in that situation.

With chronic pain, interestingly we find that the pain changes in quality, or position. Working with pain is possibly the most surprising use of EFT but, as we have seen, 'pain is in the brain' so the subjective experience of pain with its emotional overlay is what we are working on. We start by giving the pain a full description; is it dull or sharp, nagging or constant. We may even assign a colour (the subconscious mind works in metaphor and assigns symbols and associations to things – colour being one way of accessing this).

Standard EFT protocol then gets the person to create a 'set-up' statement to describe their situation in the present tense and then counter it with an acceptance statement or affirmation. This has traditionally been to counter any 'psychological reversal' (commonly understood as a pay-off[119]). To give you an example it would be "even though I have this nagging, burning pain in my left leg, I deeply and completely accept myself anyway". We then tap on certain meridian points shown below in succession, usually going through 2 rounds until we've reduced the SUD score sufficiently.

Figure 27. EFT tapping points

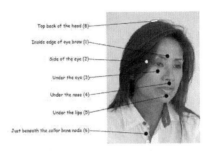

However, Robert Smith, a practitioner in the US, has developed what he calls 'Faster EFT[TM]' which does away with the set up statement formalised in this way as he maintains it is not necessary[120]. His method uses a less complicated statement which will often be standardised once the initial problem has been stated. An example would be "all this pain, this guilt, this anger, letting go". His method is more provocative, but in my experience it really is quicker, particularly if the practitioner taps on the person maintaining eye contact. It is important that the person really connects with the feelings as before, but something about acknowledging your personal pain, although difficult at first, is intensely relieving. I always say as I begin to tap "feel this for the last time" which is a very important statement both of intent and finality. This is talking the language the subconscious really understands; it's in the present and it is a clear instruction. It seems that this step is really key to what then follows which is where you pile on the agony somewhat, as you list the feelings or fears that the client has described to you. Sometimes, as a skilled therapist you will add a few of your own intuitively. This is a very different approach to standard psychotherapy which usually skirts around feelings and certainly avoids touch and contact between client and therapist. It may take a while for the uninitiated client to accept but, once they begin to feel the results as the SUD score reduces, their scepticism disappears. This stuff really works.

I once had a trial session with a lady at a show (where I was doing 20 minute taster sessions) who told me she had 'cleared all her issues years ago'; however she had chronic back pain which she wanted to work on. As we began tapping I mentioned 'letting go of guilt' and her eyes suddenly seemed those of a frightened child. I had no idea what her issues were (these psychosensory interventions can often be completely content free although I usually try and get an inkling of what is going on in order to be able to target more effectively). As long as the person having the treatment knows what the issue is, that is all you need. As we continued the tapping procedure we found that she couldn't forgive herself and that was the cause of her back pain. As we tapped it away she looked visibly relieved. She had been carrying the guilt of childhood pain, and it was trapped in her back. When she stood up, she announced her back pain was gone and when I saw her 3 weeks later it had not returned. Both she and I were surprised at the speed of resolution.

I appreciate that those of you for whom this is completely new might be reading this with incredulity. That was my position a few years ago I can assure you. How on earth can tapping on the body do this? Well, there are various theories out there but my feeling is that it somehow works via the motor cortex, to distract your conscious mind while you deliver the set-up statement to the subconscious. There are various other theories also (see below for EMDR for more discussion of this).

You might wonder if it is this effective why isn't everyone using it? Well the truth is it works better for some people than others, depending on how easily they find it to connect with their feelings (it's quite difficult with dissociated people), but it does have remarkable results, particularly with PTSD. The research literature is beginning to show good quality trials, but they are usually restricted to ex-soldiers or rape victims, with diagnosed PTSD which is very strictly measured. There is little research on milder forms of PTSD resulting from more everyday, cumulative trauma or those in chronic pain for whom trauma has been implicated. This is something I would love to rectify but conducting randomised trials as recommended as the gold standard of research is very expensive – that is why it is seldom done outside pharmaceutical research. As it needs to be randomised (there is no bias to selection) you cannot choose your own patients (who by coming to see you have self-selected). Another feature of a randomised controlled trial (RCT) is the need to establish a placebo against which to measure – you have to have the null treatment to compare it to. This is almost impossible to achieve as it is difficult to give a sham treatment of EFT – do you talk to them but not tap? Do you give 'standard treatment' (usually talking therapy?). Even if you do measure against talking therapy, the results are still impressive.

I'm sure you're wondering, if it's so effective why isn't it offered as a standard primary care option for people suffering pain, addictions, anxiety, etc? Once again I think a historical division of medicine into physical and mental with different branches of practice means that psychiatry has an inherent ignorance (and some would say bias against the body). It is not because of lack of efficacy. I can only once again urge you to try it before you decry it. Oh and read the research evidence and supportive literature - there's lots on the EFT Register[121].

Matrix Re-imprinting

Recently, there has been a further development in EFT practice which has been called Matrix Re-imprinting[122]. Invented by Karl Dawson, this takes EFT to a new dimension wherein you are taken back to a difficult time in your life that you would like to clear by 'associating' back into the person you were (your 'ECHO' as it is termed) via your imagination. By revisiting that younger internal representation of yourself you connect energetically with that 'part' of you that is stuck and helpless, offering support (via imagining tapping on him / her) and you recreate a new and different ending to the original event.

Although this may sound a little wacky to those who have not come across it before, I can report that, strange as it may seem, it genuinely has an effect on limbically-stored (implicit) memory, and de-stresses the body very effectively. In psychological terms you are clearing the memory of part of you that is still in distress and releasing the energy of maintaining that psychological defence. It is not so dissimilar to a lot of hypnotherapeutic interventions or, for that matter, those of conventional psychology. The terminology, though, may put some people off as it borrows from the recent 'new age' ideas of energy being stored in an eternal 'matrix' which we tune into. Whether or not that is true (and it is not so far-fetched as we have seen from the quantum biology of Rupert Sheldrake's morphic resonance or Jungian archetypes), it certainly has some interesting effects and is worth investigating. When I used it to clear a traumatic memory of mine, there were definitely long-lasting beneficial effects. There is some considerable research evidence beginning to come out too about its efficacy.

EMDR

This relatively new technique was discovered by psychologist Francine Shapiro whilst walking in the woods one day. As her eyes darted backwards and forwards she noticed that the emotional feelings that she was having about her health problems diminished in their upsetting effects. Being a psychotherapist, she wondered if she could replicate this in a clinical setting and she set about trying various ways of formulating the eye movements that she experienced that day. Eventually she developed a protocol which she called Eye Movement Desensitisation and Reprocessing (EMDR). Without trying to replicate the full protocol here (which can be read about in various other books, including those by Dr Shapiro and others[123,124], it is probably more useful to mention how I believe it works and how and when to use it.

There are various theories about how it works, the most possible in my opinion is connecting right and left parts of the brain, specifically the anterior cingulated cortex (ACC) so that it can come online and inhibit the amygdala responsible for fear processing. This allows the brain to begin to reprocess the memories logically so that:

The brain is able to locate the time of the event as being in the past rather than the ever present of traumatic memory, and

The brain / mind can gain insight into the beliefs that are carried with the event and challenge them

Thus for instance if, as a child, you were emotionally abused, you begin to see that it wasn't your fault, that you aren't inherently bad (no shame), what you did was a survival tool which worked but is no longer valid as an adult. You gain perspective on your parent/caretaker from an adult view and see that their participation was not your fault as the power in that situation was with the perpetrator. In situations that are less charged it is sometime possible to come to a state of acceptance as you realise what they did was often because of their own pain. Often, you are able to reach a state of forgiveness too, but initially it is enough just to realise (feel in your body) that you were not responsible for the abuse at an emotional/gut level.

The reprocessing part of the process occurs as the memory is brought out of limbic storage and adaptively processed in the normal 'memory networks' in the brain rather than stuck in emotional memory. Usually this happens within a couple of session appointments, consisting of several 'rounds' of moving the fingers back and forth in front of the eyes. EMDR is remarkably quick. I liken it to a precision instrument rather than a hammer cracking the proverbial nut.

Before the session clients are asked to fill in a form detailing their 5 most troubling memories. This may be events in their distant past or more recent ones. The practitioner takes great care to establish a safe mental space before beginning. I use havening (stroking the arms) to establish this or sometimes hypnotherapy whereby the person will imagine being in a place which they feel is safe to them and where they have been happy. We will then begin by asking the client to focus on an event that is troubling them (and this can be a silent process). I get them to go into that memory and evoke the feelings; usually this is not difficult as they have been living with these feelings just under the surface sometimes for years. Sometimes I ask them to describe the feeling with words too e.g. 'I'm alone'

I ask them where in their body they feel it and they close their eyes and find where it resides - common places are the chest, stomach and throat (these have mindbody significance to the problem too – throat is often something unspoken for instance). Once they are really focussed on the feeling, they open their eyes and we begin. I ask the client to focus on left to right passes of my fingers across their field of vision without moving their head (i.e. just with eye movement)[1]. This is very important. I watch closely as we silently work together, me moving my fingers from side to side and they watching that movement. Usually, I can see immediately when something has come into their mind as the eyes jump. Sometimes this takes a few rounds to establish, as certain personality types (type A's for instance) are still doubting that this can work and their thinking brains are running a dialogue such as "this is stupid, this won't work, how weird is this?". The next thing that may come up is they are trying to make it work (perfectly) and the concentration stops them actually going into the feeling. I usually am able to pick this up and I remind them it isn't a test and to just let whatever comes into their minds come up, without judgement. Soon enough the cognitive mind eventually lets go within a few rounds and new associations are formed.

Interestingly the things that pop up, usually with a corresponding jump in the eye movement, are the 'odd', seemingly 'random' things like an even older memory, or a person or a belief. Far from random, these events are all linked together in your emotional brain by a similar feeling and so each one that comes up is another one that needs to be cleared. What happens in EMDR is the memories and their traumatic emotional meaning are then disconnected - permanently. You still have the memory but the meaning you made of it when you were young is overwritten with something from

---

1 Some EMDR therapists substitute eye movements with alternating taps or tones; all forms of bilateral stimulation (BLS), to engage our brain's natural healing system.

an adult perspective. This immediately relieves the emotional pressure and the person is released from the energy-wasting drain of old emotions carried subconsciously. I always stress that the client is in control throughout the process and it is them doing the healing as their brain knows what it needs.

So, we work systematically from the worst memory (the 'target' – unfortunately militaristic terminology!) through to any related events where the emotion was the same until we have reduced the emotional strength (measured by a SAD score – as in EFT and other psychological treatments).

I have observed that a client's whole facial expression is visibly changed by the experience. People find it hard to believe but I watch them 'grow up' in front of me. My theory is that when people focus on an old emotional memory, they go back in their mind to the time of that event and they 'become' that younger version of themselves; their mind is re-creating that event for them, and their autonomic nervous system carries the nervous signals via the vagus nerve to various parts of their body. As we have learnt from polyvagal theory the vagus controls the face and facial expression for bonding/attachment purposes. A child that has been humiliated or shamed will show that in their face and when you re-enact that memory, the adult returns to having those feelings and the face and posture reflect this. One of the ways in which I know we've successfully 'reprocessed' that memory is that shift in posture and facial expression. It is truly remarkable.

The therapist does not intervene in ways that other therapies commonly use.. They do not question, suggest or interpret events. They only ask that the client 'go with the feeling'. If another feeling or thought comes up, we instruct them to 'follow that'. Occasionally we may interject with an 'interweave' which is an entirely organic process of following whatever the mind brings up itself. Thus it is self-directed and client-centred. It is also a mindful practice as we avoid judgement or trying to control the thought/belief. As such it falls into line with many other modern psychotherapeutic practice.

The other factor that surprises people is that the effects of EMDR don't stop when they leave my office. It is a memory reconsolidation process after all; the brain is re-wiring by taking the memory out of the limbic system to put it where it belongs into non-emotional long-term memory. What seems to happen is when you light up a new neural pathway in this manner the brain continues to do this even after the session.

I had a client who was suffering symptoms of panic attacks. We did EMDR together where we worked on a more recent trauma that she had had that was highly linked to the original trauma. She was reluctant to tell me the story as it clearly upset her a great deal. So we worked on it metaphorically – she described it as 'having lost her legs'. We did the eye movements and almost immediately visions of the event came up in lurid detail, tears came to her eyes, but I asked her to trust the process rather than avoid and we worked through the pain. Here then EMDR differs from most standard therapies that find ways to circumvent the pain rather than allowing the person to relive it for fear of re-traumatising them. This is an important consideration but with EMDR the relief is usually so quick that the trauma is felt very fleetingly and then there is release. I emphasise this by asking them to feel it 'for the last time'.

As the client began to see what had happened and how it was linked to the past beliefs she had been carrying, further revelations came one after another. She realised far from this event 'proving' that she was a failure, that in fact she had been given everything in place at that particular time to enable her to get through it and not only survive but enable her partner to survive also. She saw that it was not the disaster she had perceived which confirmed her guilt but the success which ensured her liberation. The relief and self-understanding were immediate. She said to me afterwards that life became hopeful again from that day.

As this was my first experience of using EMDR (I had only just qualified!), it remains a seminal experience for me also. I had never before found a tool with such precision and speed. I became convinced that this extraordinary technique heals people. We may not know exactly how yet (but we will), but to me that is immaterial. We are working with the mindbody, which is largely a mystery to us, though it is likely that we will find more answers very soon through continuing to develop an evidence base for the technique[125].

Applied Kinesiology – Psych-K™

Some of you may have come across kinesiology as 'muscle testing', where the therapist tests the strength of the arm muscle. It is most well known as a method used by some physical therapists such as chiropractors to check areas of physical dysfunction in the body. I was first introduced to kinesiology by a friend who wanted to demonstrate how the mind controls what nerve signals are sent to the muscles. The standard explanation is that the muscles will enable the arm to lock very effectively when the body and mind are in harmony. When they are in discord the muscles simply do not have the power. There is nothing mystical or magical about this; it is a biological / neurological fact. It is therefore a method of simple biofeedback, which has a long history of use.

There is a further development that the muscle test will indicate areas of weakness when you touch certain energy points or meridians on other parts of the body. I have had this done and it is quite clear that you feel weaker when certain points on the head and body are touched. Quite why this is so is not so easily explained but may have to do with a similar effect to EFT which taps on certain areas of the body. One could argue that, since we are surrounded by and generating electromagnetic fields, we are interacting with that. Whatever the explanation, it is a powerful means of communication with your body and has recently been used as a psychological intervention aka Psych-K[TM].

Rob Williams devised a protocol after years of struggling with his own issues and experimenting with kinesiology. He maintains that the body reads the subconscious (which I would agree with) and therefore to enable change to be instigated properly you need to check in with the subconscious via the body. He uses the body as a means of establishing communication with the mind. His protocol consists of 3 areas;

The conflict communication; when a person is asked to state something which they know to be untrue their muscles go weak. A good example would be to get someone to hold out their dominant arm (right or left handed) to the side and ask them to look at the floor with their head facing straight ahead[1] while stating their name. You then ask them to hold strong and they do their best to resist your downward pressure. People usually manage this with no problem. You then repeat but this time they state something that is patently untrue. It is good to make the statement one that is a good contrast with the previous true statement. For instance if the person is female make the name a male name so that not only is the name untrue but it reflects the wrong gender. Ask them to then repeat this statement while resisting your downward pressure. Most people go weak even though they have every intention of staying strong (just to disprove your suggestion).

The stress detector; when a person is similarly asked to maintain a strong arm whilst thinking of something you can check whether that thought is a stressful one. For instance if when you think of your mother your arm goes weak it indicates that you find that relationship a stressful one. This is despite your best intentions (willpower) or how hard you might have logically processed that issue. That is because both the strength of logic and the effort of willpower, both of which reside in the thinking brain (cortex), are far weaker than the subconscious (where the imagination

1 Eye position is important as it tends to relate to where in their mind they are representing the statement – this is a basic tenet of NLP based on studying eye movements and their relation to memory processing. With the eyes down there is more emotional engagement to what you are saying. Why is this?

resides). This is useful if you want to identify an area of weakness which might need to be re-visited within psychosensory therapy.

The communications system; we get the body to indicate whether it agrees with a statement (a variation on the first point). You firstly set up the communication by getting them to think of the word yes over and over whilst testing the arm. You then repeat with the word 'no'. In most cases the arm goes weak. Please note there should be no difference in the strength of the pressing down of the arm – you should be aware that the arm goes weak of its own accord, you are not trying to prove a point. This is not about the ego of the practitioner or the client; it is really about noticing how the body is communicating with you in a very powerful way.

The suggested protocol then tests various beliefs, getting permission at each stage with the subconscious, and then post-tests the belief once you have completed a staged protocol. Try it for yourself; belief statements that cause problems can be something like:

- I can achieve anything I chose.
- I am a worthy and competent person.
- I am intelligent and capable.
- I do my best and my best is good enough.
- I can attract money into my life and use it wisely.
- I deserve happiness and success in my life.

Havening

Havening was developed in the US by clinican /researcher Ronald R Ruden and has been further modified by TV hypnotherapist Paul McKenna in the UK[126]. It uses a combination of eye movements and touch (strokes to the arms usually) to establish a safe feeling in the body and disconnect troublesome memories from emotional content. It has been used successfully to help people overcome nightmares, cravings and other unwanted behaviour like over-eating. I use it within a hypnotherapeutic framework to ground the body prior to more in-depth work. It may be that stroking simulates the mother's cuddling of the baby when first born to stimulate bonding by priming the social engagement system and thus downregulating the lower levels of the ANS. There is a wonderful example of this online called 'the rescuing hug' with twin baby girls, one of whom instinctively hugged the other to save her life and changed the practice of neo-natal care overnight[127]. We simply do not know the myriad ways in which the mind and body interact. But we can harness it.

All these interventions are examples of energy medicine. Western medicine has not (yet) recognised the energy of the body to be a real phenomenon and so cannot imagine harnessing it. However there are some clinicians using these techniques and trying to get them recognised. In particular, Donna Eden and her clinical psychologist husband, David Feinstein, are doing a lot of fine research getting studies published to make this sort of work accepted[128]. My experience using kinesiology is that it is an excellent method to remove blocks and resistance to change.

Summary of trauma therapy

I don't claim that I have been exhaustive in my coverage of therapies that work. I have only detailed those that I use or ones I have personally experienced. What all the therapies that I use (and probably many others that I don't) have in common is that they facilitate self-acceptance and understanding via accessing feelings through the body. Research confirms that a 'felt sense' was the single variable that was the most robust for inducing change. It doesn't matter so much which type of therapy you go for (and you may find you try more than one), more important is that whatever therapy you chose references the body. It is vital that the therapist is able "to find the ways that the body experiences power and mastery"[129].

Instead of giving away power to 'experts' who take control of their 'disease/illness/issue', the person has the opportunity to look at their problem as a symptom of a wider imbalance in their life which may need addressing. Imbalance may be the essence of dis-ease. Let's not forget that our model of disease, based as it is on our nineteenth century understanding of the body as machine, may be completely wrong. Illness may not be the enemy after all; it could be seen instead as "an entirely purposeful and meaningful yet subconscious expression of an underlying disparity between innate and learned needs – a maladaptive stress response"[76].

With this model people are more able to take control for themselves and their life by seeing the precursors to the current symptoms, which will have been there all along. By going through the process with a skilled practitioner, to 'make the unconscious conscious' and reveal, like the layers of an onion, the levels of unhelpful belief and self-image that have contributed to where they are in their lives. Ultimately it is the client who heals themselves, I am merely the facilitator.

In the process clients may gain many insights, in particular self-worth. According to the work of the self-help pioneer Byron Katie, it takes only one person to change a relationship[130]. I always say "*you change yourself, you change everything.*" The relationships you have, the life experiences you have been attracting are all subtly altered when you 'defuse' the traumatic memory component. There are also many physical pay-offs; if you accept the wisdom that an underlying belief causes an unconscious activation of the stress response (which is what this book and others have argued) then it makes sense that when you release the mindbody from this, the resulting return to homeostasis means the physical body can shift from protection (fight, flight and freeze) to growth and repair. So your immune system instead of being on alert (which results in either over-activation or exhaustion) can return to being quiescent until needed, whereupon a proportionate response will result. In effect then the balance is restored and you can begin to return to the state of health you enjoyed naturally when you were a child (assuming you had reasonable health as a child). Your liver begins to detoxify better, your hormones adjust to balance properly, your heart rate is steadier, your connective tissue is able to repair, your skin, hair and eyes look brighter. Freed of its burden the body is able to heal.

The benefits of truly healing your life extend beyond the physical and go into the metaphysical. When you look at your life not as a series of random events or the result of your genetics, fate or whatever, but as a direct result of your underlying beliefs and behaviours, then you begin to take responsibility for it. This has wide ramifications for my clients and the people with whom they are in relationship.

Many people come to me with wide-ranging problems in their lives – not just chronic pain but issues with their children/spouse/boss and so on. This is not unusual in that chronic pain is often the symptom of a wider imbalance. Chrysalis Effect therapists often say "the problem is rarely the problem" meaning that what the client presents with is rarely the only, or even the main, problem. It is often a result of wider issues/ conflicts present in their lives. We are seldom challenged in our beliefs until we are in relationship with another.

I am very careful to point out that we can't 'fix' the other person but we can change the way that you respond to that situation, and in so doing, *everything* changes. Not just your level of pain, but your guilt, disappointment, resentment, rage and all the other uncomfortable feelings that you've been burying and that are largely responsible for your pain, begin to melt away as you see the old programmes you have been running and how you have created your reality. There is a very big movement in alternative circles that talks of the 'Law of Attraction'[88], a metaphysical principle whereby what you continually ask for in your subconscious mind (things you obsess and worry about) are brought to you. So, you may say, "I want to be rich and successful", but underneath the surfaceyou are running a programme which says "you'll never make anything of yourself" or "you're a failure" (often these are the voices of our parents or other significant people in our lives). This so called 'monkey-mind' of negative self-talk has the effect of colouring our perceptions of the world to the point where, in anticipation of rejection and failure for instance, we actually draw it to ourselves more.

This does have recognition within psychology as the principle of re-enactment whereby a pattern of abuse is continued into adult life. Psychologically rather than metaphysically this is a way that the mindbody is trying to somehow resolve the issue by repeating it to allow completion. But this resolution seldom happens and more often the person is further traumatised by subsequent experience. Remember that the mind is always trying to do the best for you in every situation. It may just not have the right tools for the job. Compounding the problem of having a Palaeolithic brain in a 21st century life are our modern lifestyles; where play is downgraded in favour of work, where supportive relationships are rare and usually relegated to those with our significant other (if we have one), and our external communities are fragmented and competitive, which often fails to help us process our internal dialogue.

Our problems in the wider world - war, pollution, climate change, and so on - are simply a reflection of our inner turmoil. When we no longer have any connection with our deeper self, we lose touch with each other and with our planet. We desperately need to re-connect to our purpose and value, to find meaning in our work and relationships. We cannot do that when we are for all intents and purposes 'asleep' in our lives. Most of us are going through the motions of living fruitful lives with the attendant rewards; money, possessions, status, and so on without actually feeling connected to any of it at a spiritual level. Of course we have moments of joy - the birth of our children, a hard-won achievement, recovery from illness and so on - but they are few and far between. What I aim to do for myself and all the people I work with is to find joy in the everyday, free of trauma and unresolved emotion. For this is really living. I don't want to give people unreasonable expectations of a 'quick fix' as that is not what this is about. This is about process, self-exploration and knowledge. It can be painful and difficult, but the rewards are immense. I'm not there yet by the way, but I'm on the road. I hope you'll join me.

EPILOGUE

Whilst writing this book a number of events forced me to evaluate further the effects of trauma on the body. The first was the illness of my elderly mother which necessitated a complete review of my relationship to her. I did not feel impelled to tell her about the book; I think she would have found it upsetting and I did not wish to add to her burden. However, in writing it, a catharsis of sorts awaited me. I began to be aware of my extreme hyper-responsibility towards my Mum and it began to give me symptoms of hormonal distress. However, due to a synchronicity of events (including revelatory dreams, chance meetings with key people, and extraordinary information which I uncovered and energetic interventions I undertook) I was led to some further healing myself which has made this book both a professional and personal odyssey.

It shows me that our learning never stops. Indeed I have determined that this book be the basis of some further training for me. I am now undertaking a PhD in which I look forward to revealing more about myself and others' responses to the events of our lives.

CREDITS

Thanks to all the people, clients, family and friends who have helped me on this journey of discovery. I look forward to meeting many more of you, the adventurers out there. Although I have no idea who you are yet, I know that you're there and in writing this book I aim to connect with you. I am certain of one thing; we need to move away from our culture of fear and step into love – of ourselves, each other and our planet131.When we embrace wellness as a way of living rather than waiting for disease to catch up with us, we are empowered to live wholeheartedly. For that is what we need to do if we are to move forward out of the current paradigm of health to a new awakening.

FURTHER READING

Books

James Alexander, *The Hidden Psychology of Pain*. A very accessible book for sufferers and practitioners which explains in great detail how the psychology of pain perpetuates it.
Aron, Elaine N. *The Highly Sensitive Person*. Element. A fantastic book written in easy to understand language about how hypersensitivity affects people throughout life. Although not explicitly a book about trauma, it covers the

same ground.

Brene Brown: *Daring Greatly*: How the Courage to Be Vulnerable Transforms the Way We Live, Love, Parent, and Lead. About the way shame invades our culture and what makes you shame resilient.

David Hamilton The Mindbody Bible

David Hanscom. *Back in Control*. A spine surgeon's account of recovering from back pain via emotional resolution and away from surgical treatments. Compelling.

Bessel Van der Kolk: The *Body Keeps the Score*. With a long career in trauma rehabilitation and treatment, this is the absolute bible for trauma treatment

Peter Levine; *Healing Trauma* and *Chasing the Tiger*. Both classics which show how an uncompleted freeze response may lie behind the chronic symptoms of trauma.

Bruce Lipton *The Biology of Belief*. One of the first books to explain epigenetics i.e. the effect of the environment on the genetic expression of DNA. A must read.

Gabor Mate; *When the Body says no*. A lay person's book which aims to outline what stress does and how it works.

Sarah Myhill: *Diagnosis and Treatment of CFS*; it's mitochondria not hypochondria. One of the most comprehensive books on the mitochondrial causation of CFS and how Dr Myhill's clinic treats it. She was one of the pioneers in this field and lost her licence to practice as a GP because of it. She now operates privately.

Pat Ogden, *Trauma and the Body* - wonderful information about how trauma can be overcome. Primarily for practitioners. Developer of Somatic Sensing™.

Georgie Oldfield, Chronic Pain; your Key to Recovery – this book comes from someone working in a similar way to me which follows the work of Sarno. From physical to emotional recovery.

Daniel Siegel: *Mindsight: Change your Brain and your Life*. Excellent book for the lay person on how to change your mind's 'maps of the world' with specific exercises and case studies.

Robert Scaer, *The Body Bears the Burden*. Another really great book which looks in detail at the neurobiology of trauma and how it translates into damage to brain and body.

Francine Shapiro. *Getting Past your past*. A book on EMDR technique for the layperson

Dr Dave Clarke They can't find anything wrong

Dr Howard Schubiner Unlearn your pain

Websites

http://www.alchemytherapies.co.uk – my website where I outline my approach and treatments

http://www.fastereft.com/ - Faster EFT is a protocol developed by Robert P Smith. Recommended

http://www.traumahealing.org/ - site devoted to Peter Levine's Somatic Experiencing modality

http://www.khironhouse.com/ Khiron house Trauma centre in the UK

http://www.janinafisher.com/ training in trauma therapy

http://www.thechrysaliseffect.com/ training in Chronic fatigue related syndromes

http://www.drdansiegel.com/ training in interpersonal neurobiology or 'mindsight'.

http://www.drirind,com all about thyroid and adrenal insufficiency

http://www.sirpauk.com   SIRPA – Pain Relief and Recovery organisation in the UK based on Dr Sarno's work

http://www.traumacenter.org/ Bessel van der Kolk's US Institute

http://www.emdr.com/ Francine Shapiro's EMDR institute

ABOUT THE AUTHOR

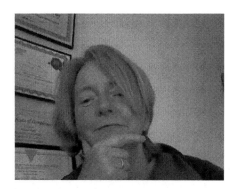

Patricia Worby, BSc. MSc. is a former scientist, now researcher and specialist practitioner in chronic fatigue and pain . She worked for the NHS for 15 years and currently the University of Southampton for 10 years in clinical research and latterly as a Research Manager. After graduation she was going to 'change the world through science' but life intervened in a quite surprising way.

After a series of health challenges in her 30's, including depression and chronic fatigue, she was encouraged to find her own answers and is now a passionate advocate of natural medicine. Today, she is a holistic therapist who specialises in chronic illness especially ME/CFS and Fibromyalgia using nutrition, massage and emotional healing. She is currently undertaking a PhD in the links between implicit memory and chronic pain..

She can be found online at www.alchemytherapies.co.uk.

[1] Levine, Peter. (2008) *Healing Trauma*. Sounds True.

[2] Peter Levine, (1997) *Waking the Tiger* North Atlantic Books.

[3] Mol SS et al. (2005). Symptoms of post-traumatic stress disorder after non-traumatic events: evidence from an open population study. *Br J Psychiatry*, 186(6):494–9

4 Cvetek R. (2008). EMDR treatment of distressful experiences that fail to meet the criteria for PTSD. *J. EMDR Practice and Research*, 2(1):2–14

5 Alexander, James (2012) *The Hidden Psychology of Pain*, Balboa Press P 195

6 Sabrina Weyeneth http://sabrinaweyeneth.com/

7 Brown, Brené, *The Power of Vulnerability* talks on www.udemy.com/the-power-of-vulnerability

8 Levine, Peter. in http://www.psychotherapy.net/interview/interview-peter-levine

9 Price, Weston.(2009). *Nutrition and Physical Degeneration*. Price Pottenger Nutrition

10 Brene Brown.(2012). *Daring Greatly*. Portfolio Penguin.

11 Panskepp Jaak and Biven, Lucy. (2012) *The Archaeology of Mind*. Norton.

12 The Chrysalis Effect Practitioner training www.thechrysaliseffect.com

13 Skull, Andrew.(2013) in the Lancet quoted in review of *'Cracked; Why Psychiatry is Doing More Harm Than Good* by James Davies, Icon Books

14 Candace Pert (1999) *The molecules of emotion*.

15 Siegel, Daniel (2013) from the introduction to Pat Ogden *Trauma and the body*

16 Gabor Mate (2013); *When the Body says No*. Wiley.

17 Pizzorno Joe. (2000) *Encyclopaedia of Natural Healing*. Sphere.

18 Hadhazy, Adam.(2010). Think Twice: How the Gut's "Second Brain" Influences Mood and Well-Being. *Scientific American*. February 12

19 Yatsunenko, et al. (2012). Human gut microbiome viewed across age and geography. *Nature*, 48 6(7402), 222–227. doi:10.1038/nature11053

20 The Human Microbiome: considerations for pregnancy, birth and early mothering. January 2015 http://midwifethinking.com/2014/01/15

21 D'Angelis Tore, (2002) *A bright future for PNI*, APA.

22 Maier et al.(1998) The role of the vagus nerve in cytokine-to-brain communication. *Ann. New York Acad Sciences* http://www.ncbi.nlm.nih.gov/pubmed/ 9629257

23 Robert Scaer, (2014) *The Body Bears the Burden*,

24 Galland , Leo.(2014) *The Gut Microbiome and the Brain*. Foundation for Integrated Medicine, New York.

25 Moorjani, Anita (2012) *Dying to be Me,* Hay House.

26 Panksepp, J Biven L, (2012) *The Archaeology of Mind,* Norton P309

27 Maclean, P. (1989). *The Triune Brain in Evolution.* Plenum. New York.

28 Van der Kolk, Bessel from the introduction to Pat Ogden (2006). *Trauma and the body.* Norton.

29 Etymology online http://www.etymonline.com/index.php?term=emotion

30 Sperry, Roger who won the Nobel Prize for medicine in 1981, quoted in Pat Ogden Trauma and the body, 2013

31 Llinás, Rodolfo.(2001). *I of the Vortex: From Neurons to Self.* The MIT Press,

32 van der Kolk, Bessel. Dissociation, Affect Dysregulation & Somatization. *American Journal of Psychiatry,* 153(7) 1996

33 Seligman, Martin P. (2006) *Learned optimism; learn to change your mind and your life.* Vintage Books.

34 Ogden, Pat.(2006) *Trauma and the Body* p81

35 Shore, Allan.(2003). Affect *Dysregulation and Disorders of the Self.* Norton.

36 Lyons-Ruth (2000) from Janina Fisher trauma training 2015

37 Chitty, John. www.energyschool.com from Chapter Six in "Dancing with Yin and Yang" CSES.

38 Tyrell Ivan & Griffin, Joe. (2007). *How to Master Anxiety,* Human Givens Books.

39 LeDoux, Joseph. (2002). *The synaptic self: how our brains become who we are.* New York: Guilford Press.

40 Glenville, Marilyn, (2006). *Fat around the middle.* Kyle Cathie.

41 McCraty Rollin and Zayas (2014). Cardiac coherence, self-regulation, autonomic stability, and psychosocial well-being *Front. Psychol.,* 29 September

42 McGonical, Kelly. *How to make stress your friend.* TED talk http://www.ted.com/talks/kelly_mcgonigal_how_to_make_stress_your_friend?language=enl

43 Institute of HeartMath. http://www.heartmath.org/research/research-home/heart-rate-variability.html

44 McCraty, et al (2004). Electrophysiological evidence of intuition: part 1. The surprising role of the heart *J. Altern Complement Med.* Feb;10(1):133-143

45 Salem Mohammed Omar, Prof. *The Heart, Mind and Spirit* accessed at https://www.rcpsych.ac.uk/pdf/Heart,%20Mind%20and%20Spirit%20%20Mohamed%20Salem.pdf

46 Crowther, Gillian, (2015).The secrets of Mitochondrial Information

Transfer; implications for health and disease, CAM Seminar see www.aonm.com

47 Xu Chen, et al. (2014) Light-harvesting chlorophyll pigments enable mammalian mitochondria to capture photonic energy and produce ATP. *J. Cell Science* 127, 388–399

48 Crawford, M et al. A quantum theory for the irreplaceable role of docosahexaenoic acid in neural cell signalling throughout evolution. *Prostaglandins, Leukotrienes and Essential Fatty Acids*, 88:1

49 Berg JM et al. (2011) *Biochemistry* 7th Edition. NY.

50 Naviaux, R.K.(2014). Metabolic features of the cell danger response. *Mitochondrion* May;16:7-17

51 Wren, Barbara.(2009). Cellular awakening; how your body holds and creates Light.

52 Lipton, Bruce.(2011). *The Biology of Belief,* Hay House.

53 Arden, D John. (2010). *Rewire your brain*, Wiley.

54 Shore, Allan. *Attachment and the regulation of the right brain* http://www.allanschore.com/pdf / SchoreAttachHumDev.pdf

55 Taylor, Graeme. Quoted in Allan Schore, Affect Regulation and the Origin of the Self: *The Neurobiology of Emotional Development* P440

56 Ebner K1, Singewald N. (2006). The role of substance P in stress and anxiety responses. *Amino Acids.* 31(3):251-72.

57 Alexander, James. (2014). The *Hidden Psychology of Pain.* Balboa Press.

58 Fischer, Janina. Trauma Therapy training. See www.janinafischer.com

59 Bergman, U. (2012). *Neurobiological Foundations for EMDR Practice* P43.

60 Meyer-Williams Linda. (1994). Recall of Childhood Trauma, *J. Consulting and Clinical Psychology* 62, 6,1167-1176

61 Brain Basics: Understanding Sleep http://www.ninds.nih.gov /disorders/ brain_basics/ understanding_sleep.htm

62 Vyazovskiy V. and Delogu A.. NREM and REM Sleep. Complementary Roles in Recovery after Wakefulness http://nro.sagepub.com/content/early/2014/03/03/1073858413518152.full.html

63 Ackermann S, Rasch B (2014). Differential effects of non-REM and REM sleep on memory consolidation. *Curr.Neurological Neuosci*, Rep Feb

64 Van der Kolk, Bessel. *The Body keeps the Score*; Allen Lane. 2015

65 Williams, Rob *The Psychology of Change*, 2011 on https://www.youtube.com/watch?v=28Tbwe_aeK4

66 Frank Sulloway quoted in Dr Janina Fisher's information on personality types. http://www.khironhouse.com/blog/character-strategies-dr-janina-

fishers-insights/
67 http://www.newmedicine.ca/german-new-medicine.php
68 Le Doux, Joseph (1994) Emotion, memory and the brain. *Sci American 270:50-57*
69 Siegel, Daniel (2012) *Mindsight; the new science of personal transformation*
70 Schubiner, Howard (2010) *Unlearn your Pain*. A 28 day process to reprogram your Brain.
71 Hay, Louise. (2004). *Heal your Life*. Hay House
72 Bergman Uri, (2012) The *Neurobiological Foundations for EMDR practice*, Chapter 8 Springer
73 Myhill, S. (2014) *Diagnosis and Treatment of Chronic Fatigue Syndrome*,
74 Chrysalis Effect Practitioner Training, The Chrysalis Effect. www.chrysaliseffect.com
75 Action for ME quoting the latest CDC data from Georgia US. http://www.actionforme.org.uk/get-informed/publications/interaction-magazine/read-selected-ia-articles/what-is-me/how-common-is-me
76 Al-Kashi, Adam in the *Introduction to Recovery* by Georgie Odlfield.
77 Oldfield, Georgie. (2012) *Chronic Pain: your key to recovery*.
78 http://www.paintoolkit.org/ An online self-help resource for people in chronic (persistent) pain.
79 https://en.wikiquote.org/wiki/V%C3%A1clav_Havel
80 Dr Rind. http://www.drrind.com/therapies/thyroid-scale
81 Lam, M and D. (2012). Natural *Therapeutics to Adrenal Fatigue Syndrome*: Proper Use of Vitamins, Glandulars, Herbs, and Hormones.
82 Wilson, James. (2002) *Adrenal Fatigue: The 21st Century Stress Syndrome*, Smart publications.
83 The Chrysalis Effect – www.thechrysaliseffect.com
84 James Gallagher Health editor, 10 December 2014 BBC News website http://www.bbc.co.uk/news/health-30411246
85 Kirsch I, et al. (2008). Initial severity and antidepressant benefits: a meta-analysis of data submitted to the Food and Drug Administration. *PLoS Med*
86 Panksepp, Jaak and Biven, Lucy. (2012) 'The *Archaeology of the Mind* P337
87 Alexander, James (2012) *The Hidden Psychology of Pain*, Balboa Press P196
88 Hicks, Ester and Jerry (2007). *The Law of Attraction* Hay House UK
89 Yapko, Michael D. (2013). *Hypnosis and Treating Depression: Applications in Clinical Practice*,
90 Cuddy, Amy. http://www.ted.com/talks/amy_cuddy_your_body_language_shapes_who_you_are?language=en
91 Oldfield, Georgie (2012) Chronic *Pain; your Key to Recovery*

92 Aron, Elaine N. (2003) *The Highly Sensitive Person* P35. Element.

93 International Society of Trauma and Dissociation (ISTD) as quoted in Trauma Dissociation and Recovery by Carolyn spring (seminar on 16/7/15 in London organised by PODS

94 Lipton, Bruce and Williams Rob. *The Biology of Perception* https://www.youtube.com/watch?v=MeZL72IStGo

95 Adams, Alison. Rejection and the Spleen. http://www.thenaturalrecoveryplan.com/articles/ Rejection-and-the-Spleen.html

96 Van der Kolk, Bessel (2011) in the foreword to *The Polyvagal Theory* by Stephen Porges,

97 Ehlert, U. (2013) Enduring psychobiological effects of childhood adversity *Psychoneuroendocrinology* Sep; 38(9):1850-7.

98 Myers Brent and Greenwood-Van Meerveld, Beverley. (2009) Role of anxiety in the pathophysiology of irritable bowel syndrome: importance of the amygdala. *Front. Neurosci.*, 10 June

99 Wikipedia https://en.wikipedia.org/wiki/Otalgia

100 Zenner et al (2006) Tinnitus sensitization: Sensory and psychophysiological aspects of a new pathway of acquired centralization of chronic tinnitus. *Otol Neurotol.* 27(8):1054-63.

101 van der Kolk Bessel, (1989) The compulsion to repeat the trauma. Re-enactment, revictimization, and masochism.1. *Psychiatr Clin North Am.* 12(2):389-411.

102 Sheldrake, Rupert. (2012) *The Science Delusion.* Coronet.

103 Tolle, Eckhart. (2001). *The Power of Now A Guide to Spiritual Enlightenment*

104 Sheldrake, Rupert. http://www.sheldrake.org/research/the-credit-crunch-for-materialism

105 Basbaum, Allan *The Science of Pain*, University of California - see www.youtube.com/watch?v=-TN1r25wAoI and *The Brain and Pain* www.youtube.com/watch?v=gQS0tdIbJ0w

106 Van der Kolk Quoted in http://www.nytimes.com/2014/05/25/magazine/a-revolutionary-approach-to-treating-ptsd.html?_r=0

107 http://www.khironhouse.com/blog/the-original-matrix-finding-our-way-back-to-a-state-of-balance/

108 Richardson J. et al. (2006). Hypnosis for procedure-related pain and distress in pediatric cancer patients: a systematic review of effectiveness and methodology related to hypnosis interventions. *J Pain Symptom Manage.* Jan;31(1):70-84

109 Aron, Elaine N. (1999). *The Highly Sensitive Person; How to Thrive When the World Overwhelms You*. Thorsons

110 Perry, Bruce D. (2009). Examining Child Maltreatment Through a Neurodevelopmental Lens: Clinical Applications of the Neurosequential Model of Therapeutics. *J. Loss and Trauma*, 14:240–255,

111 Chaitow, Leon. (2013). Fascia's function: Classical osteopathic perspectives and current research compared *J. Bodywork Movement Therapies*. 17:(3) 355

112 Myers, Thomas. (2013*) Anatomy Trains*. Churchill Livingstone see also www.anatomytrains.com/

113 Hicks MR et al, (2012). Mechanical strain applied to human fibroblasts differentially regulates skeletal myoblast differentiation. *J Appl Physiol* 113(3):465-72

114 Cicchitti L et al, (2015) Chronic inflammatory disease and osteopathy: a systematic review. *PLoS One*. 17;10(3):

115 http://www.bbc.co.uk/news/blogs-ouch-30534749

116 Feinstein, D. (2012). Acupoint Stimulation in Treating Psychological Disorders: Evidence of Efficacy. *Review of General Psychology*, 16(4), 364-380

117 http://www.eftuniverse.com/research-and-studies/eft-research

118 Murphy, Brendan. (2013). The promise of Energy Psychology Methods, http://changeahead.biz/uploads/files/EnergyPsychology-Nexus.pdf August/September

119 http://www.aliceboyes.com/behaviour-patterns/

120 Smith, Robert . Faster EFT protocol and videos on you tube.

121 EFT Register on www.eftregister.com

122 Dawson, Karl (2012). *Matrix Reimprinting using EFT:* Rewrite Your Past, Transform Your Future

123 Shapiro, Francine (2001). *EMDR Basic Principles and Practice*

124 Shapiro, Francine (2013). *Getting Past your Past*. Rodale

125 For the latest research see www.emdr.com/gpyp

126 McKenna, Paul. (2014) *Freedom From Emotional Eating* Bantam Press

127 http://consciouslifenews.com/the-rescuing-hug-and-power-of-emotions/113772/

128 Eden Donna and Feinstein, John.(2008). *Energy Medicine: How to use your body's energies for optimum health and vitality*

129 Eugene Gendlin, Focusing quoted in Dr Janina Fisher on www.khironhouse.com blog

130 Katie, Byron.(2005). *I Need Your Love - Is That True?*: How to find all the love, approval and appreciation you ever wanted. Rider.

131 Marianne Williamson, (2009). *Return to Love.*

47351111R00122

Made in the USA
Charleston, SC
09 October 2015